EMPIRE OF CARE

American Encounters / Global Interactions

A series edited by Gilbert M. Joseph and Emily S. Rosenberg

This series aims to stimulate critical perspectives and fresh interpretive frameworks for scholarship on the history of the imposing global presence of the United States. Its primary concerns include the deployment and contestation of power, the construction and deconstruction of cultural and political borders, the fluid meanings of intercultural encounters, and the complex interplay between the global and the local. American Encounters seeks to strengthen dialogue and collaboration between historians of U.S. international relations and area studies specialists.

The series encourages scholarship based on multiarchival historical research. At the same time, it supports a recognition of the representational character of all stories about the past and promotes critical inquiry into issues of subjectivity and narrative. In the process, American Encounters strives to understand the context in which meanings related to nations, cultures, and political economy are continually produced, challenged, and reshaped.

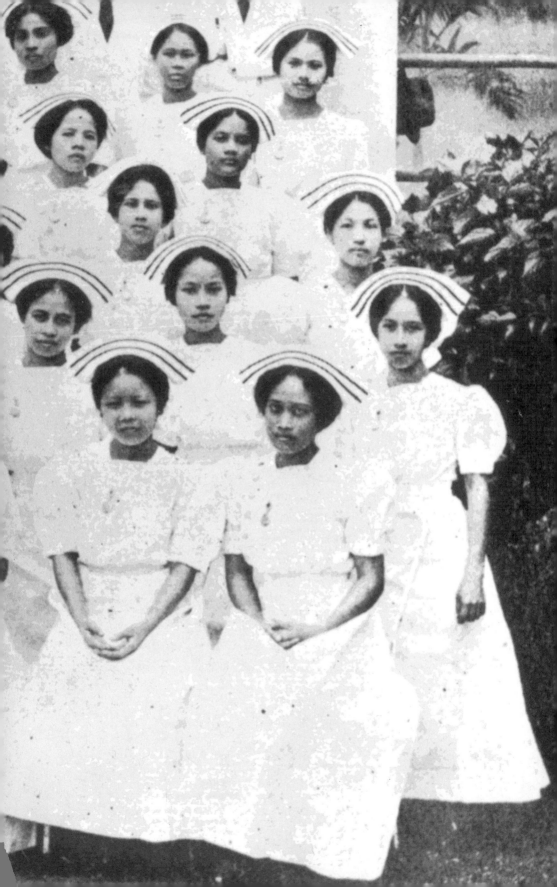

CATHERINE CENIZA CHOY

Empire of Care

Nursing and Migration in Filipino American History

DUKE UNIVERSITY PRESS   Durham and London   2003

Fifth printing, 2006

© 2003 Duke University Press

Printed in the United States of

America on acid-free paper ∞

Designed by C.H. Westmoreland

Typeset in Carter & Cone Galliard by

Keystone Typsetting, Inc.

Library of Congress Cataloging-in

Publication Data appear on the last

printed page of this book.

This book is dedicated

to my mother, Patria Ceniza,

for her loving support.

CONTENTS

ACKNOWLEDGMENTS

One of my most vivid memories of the research process for this book took place in my aunt's apartment in New York City. The apartment was typically abuzz with the conversations of elders, adults, and children because it was the main gathering place for my family to have dinner, play Bingo, watch TV, and so on. However, it also happened to be the most convenient place to interview a Filipino nurse one evening. So that evening, my *Lolo* Braulio Ceniza, *Lola* Soledad Ceniza, "Auntie" Mary Hernandez, aunts Lucy Ceniza and Vicky Paragas, cousin Brian Paragas, and my mother patiently and quietly waited in a bedroom as I interviewed the nurse in the living room for over two hours. Although the interview went well, I felt bad for inconveniencing my family. However, when the interview was finally over, they emerged from the bedroom smiling, offering the nurse something to eat, and talking excitedly and proudly about the project. For me, this experience exemplifies the ways in which my research was inextricably linked to family and community support, and challenges the notion that this book is a product of individual merit.

The many solitary hours I spent in front of a computer writing this book belie the collective nature of this project, which the cooperation, encouragement, and support from numerous individuals and groups in the United States and the Philippines have enabled. This project began as a dissertation in UCLA's History Department, where I was privileged to work with Valerie Matsumoto, Michael Salman, and Karen Brodkin, whose mentorship and scholarship I have humbly tried to emulate and from whom I continue to seek guidance.

In more recent years, the camaraderie of my colleagues Brenda Child, Rod Ferguson, Elaine Tyler May, Lary May, Carol Miller, David Noble, Jeanie O'Brien, Jennifer Pierce, Riv-Ellen Prell, and Gayle Graham Yates in the Department of American Studies at the University of Minnesota nurtured the development of this project into a book. I am especially grateful for their protection of my time during a year of research leave. My two faculty mentors, Elaine Tyler May and Josephine Lee, have been role models in every sense of the word, providing me with crucial insights for balancing scholarship, pedagogy, and family life.

When I first approached Duke University Press, I was fortunate to meet Ken Wissoker and I continue to be grateful for his enthusiasm for this project. Editors Valerie Millholland and Richard Morrison and assistant editor Miriam Angress skillfully guided this project throughout the editorial process. Natalie Kozin and Kay Robin Alexander helped me with securing the book's illustrations and permissions. Two anonymous readers provided constructive feedback that greatly informed and improved the book.

This two-shores project depended on the cooperation and support of many individuals on both sides of the ocean. In the Philippines, the nursing faculty and students at Trinity College (formerly St. Luke's Hospital) School of Nursing welcomed me in their classrooms and libraries. Dean Fe Alcantara personally introduced me to deans of other nursing schools in Manila, professional nursing leaders, and hospital supervisors.

In the United States, I am indebted to the generosity of the forty-three Filipino nurses who shared their life stories with me. Between the time of my interviews and the writing of this book, two of these nurses, Purita Asperilla and Ofelia Boado, passed away. It is my hope that this book contributes to the preservation of their memory.

Phoebe Cabotaje-Andes, Tania Azores, Lolita Compas, Maria Couper, Enrique de la Cruz, Sue Englander, Carmen Galang, Filipinas Lowery, and Mila Velasquez shared personal collections of written material when no central archive about Filipino nurses and their histories existed. Dorothy and Fred Cordova located important documents about Filipino nurses in their Filipino American National Historical Society archives. My research assistants, Karla Erickson and Felicity Schaeffer, diligently helped me organize and sort through numerous secondary and primary materials.

Rick Bonus, John Cheng, Jigna Desai, Yen Le Espiritu, Deena Gonzalez, Erika Lee, Patrick McNamara, Vicente Rafael, David Roediger, Nayan Shah, Benjamin Tolosa, Helen Toribio, and Liping Wang provided insightful comments, suggestions, and questions at conferences, lectures, and other readings that strengthened the manuscript. I am grateful to Vicente Rafael for suggesting "Empire of Care" as the title of this book.

Several funding agencies and organizations supported the research and writing of this project. A Ford Foundation Postdoctoral Fellowship administered by the National Research Council and a University of Minnesota College of Liberal Arts National Fellowship Supplement provided an invaluable year of research leave to revise the book manuscript. John Kuo Wei Tchen graciously hosted my fellowship tenure at New York University's Asian/Pacific/American Studies Program and Institute. A Grant-in-Aid for Research, Artistry, and Scholarship, a McKnight Summer Fellowship for the Arts and Humanities, and a President's Faculty Multicultural Research Award from various offices at the University of Minnesota, such as the Office of the Vice President for Research and Dean of the Graduate School, enabled research travel and other assistance for the later stages of the project. In its earlier stages, fellowships and grants from the Social Science Research Council's International Migration Program, Academy for Educational Development, UCLA's Institute of American Cultures and Center for the Study of Women, and the Consortium for a Strong Minority Presence at Liberal Arts Colleges' Minority Scholar-in-Residence Program at Pomona College provided crucial financial support.

An earlier version of sections in Chapters 1 and 2 appeared as "The Usual Subjects: Medicine, Nursing, and American Colonialism in the Philippines" in the spring 1998 issue of *Critical Mass: A Journal of Asian American Cultural Criticism*. An earlier version of sections in Chapters 1, 2, 3, and 4 appeared as "'Exported to Care': A Transnational History of Filipino Nurse Migration to the United States," in Nancy Foner, Rubén G. Rumbaut, and Steven J. Gold, eds., *Immigration Research for a New Century: Multidisciplinary Perspectives* (New York: Russell Sage Foundation, 2000). An earlier version of Chapter 3 was originally published in Josephine Lee, Imogene Lim, and Yuko Matsukawa, eds., *Re/collecting Early Asian America: Readings in Cultural History* (Philadelphia: Temple University Press, 2002) as "From Exchange Visitor to Permanent Resident: Reconsidering Filipino Nurse Migration as a Post-1965 Phenomenon." I thank the editors and the anonymous readers for their thoughtful comments and suggestions.

I wish to express my deep appreciation for the mentorship of George Sánchez, Tania Azores, and Barbara Posadas, especially during the early stages of my graduate career. In addition to the friends I have already mentioned, the friendship of Miroslava Chavez-Garcia, Yun Won Cho, Arleen Devera, Emily Lawsin, Linda Maram, Margaret Faye, Keri Hom, Maxwell Leung, Paul Simon, Traise Yamamoto, Karin Aguilar-San Juan, Mark Buccella, Kevin Kinneavy, and Walt Jacobs sustained me during the ups and downs of research and writing.

My family contributed to this book in so many valuable ways that are impossible to express fully with words. My husband, Gregory Paul Choy, contributed many important insights to this project. I am especially grateful for his day-to-day efforts to keep me, as well as this project, going. In addition to his intellectual companionship, sense of humor, and equal share in childrearing, his fabulous meals made even my bad writing days seem good. During the process of writing this book, our two bundles of Ceniza-Choy joy, Maya Kimberly and Louis Carlos, were born. I thank them for the many hours of Lego-playing, *Good Night Moon*–reading, and "The Wheels on the Bus"–singing, which in all seriousness (and fun!) contributed to the completion of the book. They, more than anyone, have literally brought home for me the important lesson that it is not obsessing with the past that matters, but understanding it in ways that may improve and enrich our present and future.

As my appendix on sources and the introduction to these acknowledgments reveal, my immediate and extended family in New York City played a tremendous role in supporting this project. My sister Caroline Ceniza-Levine patiently listened to the joys and frustrations of its progress over many long-distance phone calls and offered inspiring words of encouragement. She is truly wise beyond her years.

Finally, I dedicate this book to my mother, Patria Ceniza. Partly because of the ubiquity of the Filipino nurse in the United States and because of the book's subject matter, many people assumed that she herself is a nurse. While her own personal history as a post-1965 Filipino immigrant certainly informed the scholarly choices I made about research topics, her professional background is in accounting. I dedicate this book to her for all the times that she has confronted a Filipino friend who asked her incredulously, "What is Cathy going to do with a major in history?" I dedicate this book to her for all the times she has responded to such questions with pride about my passion for historical research. There is no word to describe the unconditional support from my immediate and extended family other than love. I am deeply humbled by it and forever grateful.

The Contours of a

Filipino American History

This book examines the unique and dynamic relationship between the professionalization of nursing and the twentieth-century migrations of Filipinos to the United States. Specifically, it analyzes the creation of an international Filipino professional nurse labor force primarily in the historical context of U.S. imperialism. In doing so, it asks us to reevaluate our most cherished cultural associations and assumptions about nursing (in particular, women's selfless and seemingly innate ability to care) as well as U.S. immigration (such as the inevitable assimilation of all immigrants) by acknowledging the complicated histories of nursing's role in U.S. colonialism and the racialization of Filipinos in the United States. It is my hope that this project helps us to confront the continuing legacies of U.S. imperialism as well as to better understand the dynamics of contemporary U.S. migration and labor.

In U.S. hospitals today, nursing is no longer exclusively practiced by white and black women in white uniforms. Between 1965 and 1988, more than seventy thousand foreign nurses entered the United States, the majority coming from Asia. Although Korea, India, and Taiwan are among the top Asian sending countries, the Philippines is by far the leading supplier of nurses to the United States.[1]

The late 1960s marked the beginnings of a profound racial and ethnic transformation of the foreign-trained nursing labor force in the United States when the increasing migrations of Filipino nurses ended decades of numerical domination by foreign-trained nurses from European countries and Canada. Paul Ong and Tania Azores estimate that at least twenty-five thousand Filipino nurses migrated to the United States between 1966 and 1985. They go so far as to suggest that in the United States "it could be argued that a discussion of immigrant Asian nurses, indeed of foreign-trained nurses in general, is predominantly about Filipino nurses."[2] By 1989, Filipino nurses comprised the overwhelming majority (73 percent) of foreign nurse graduates in the United States, and Canadian nurses comprised the second largest group (12 percent).[3]

Filipino nurses provide a critical source of labor for large metropolitan and public hospitals primarily in the states of New York, New Jersey, California, Texas, Florida, and Massachusetts.[4] In New York City, Filipinos comprise 18 percent of RN (registered nurse) staff in the city's hospitals.[5] Filipino nurses are also geographically clustered in Midwestern urban areas, in particular Chicago.[6]

Although the United States has been the leading destination for Filipino nurse migrants historically and its early twentieth-century colonial relationship with the Philippines distinguishes it from other receiving countries of Filipino nurse migrants, the international migration of Filipino nurses is inextricably linked to the larger processes of global restructuring in which the increased demands for services in highly developed countries as well as the export of manufacturing to developing countries have contributed to increasing worldwide mobility. In 1979, the authors of a World Health Organization report observed that the geographical distribution of the international migration of nurses was highly imbalanced.[7] Of an estimated fifteen thousand nurses moving each year, over 90 percent went to eight countries, mainly to the United States, the United Kingdom, and Canada. The authors also observed that, among the nurse-sending countries, the largest outflow of nurses "by far" was from the Philippines.

These observations suggest that, first, the phenomenon of Filipino nurse migration to the United States is only one window from which to view the global dimensions of this predominantly female gendered migrant flow that emanates from the Philippines. As James Tyner points out, "Whereas early Philippine immigration consisted predominantly of male laborers to the United States, current flows are directed to more than 130 countries, each revealing distinctive sex differences in composition."[8] Second, although the WHO report's observations might be read in a celebratory way that speaks to the ability of the nurses' highly skilled training to cross national and cultural borders, it also illustrates how these professional migration flows are embedded in a global structure of power in which nurses from countries with comparatively even higher nursing shortages are migrating to provide professional nursing care for populations of primarily highly developed countries such as the United States, Canada, and the United Kingdom. According to the WHO report, "Nurses are even more inequitably distributed around the world than are physicians."[9] When two-thirds of the world's population living in developing countries have only a small fraction, 15 percent, of the world's nurses, international nurse migration patterns only exacerbate these inequalities of health services, inequalities that I refer to as an "empire of care."

Despite the important role that Filipino nurse migrants play in the United States and other countries, we know little about the development of this phenomenon as well as the nurse migrants themselves. Although renewed interest in the migration of highly trained persons to the United States has produced a number of studies that have *included* Filipino nurse migrants, these studies often lump them together with flows of other Asian professional migrants.[10] These studies provide valuable information about the national origins and highly skilled nature of contemporary migration patterns to the United States, but the lumping of Filipino nurse migrants with professional migrants from other Asian sending countries and/or other professional migrants from the Philippines produces some troubling effects. First, it tends to foreground the uniqueness of the United States as a receiving nation of a diverse group of highly skilled migrants. Many of these studies generally refer to contemporary U.S. immigration legislation and economic opportunities to explain the phenomenon of Filipino nurse migration. In particular, they highlight the 1965 U.S. Immigration Act's new visas allocated to workers with needed skills and critical U.S. nursing shortages in the post–World War II period. Second, although some studies have emphasized the unique situations of the Asian countries that send professional migrants, they continue to emphasize an economic logic to explain professional migration, often referred to as "brain drain." These studies argue that the inability of Asian countries to provide professional and economic opportunities to their professionals commensurate with their skills and training combined with economic opportunities in the United States produce these professional migrant flows.[11] Third, the statistical nature of these studies renders Filipino nurse migrants impersonal, faceless objects of study, an objectification that prevents an understanding and appreciation of these migrants as multidimensional historical agents, and consequently hinders an identification with them as professionals, women, and immigrants.

I characterize these effects as troubling because the emphasis on U.S.

immigration legislation and economic opportunities reinscribes the popular notion that these contemporary Filipino nurse migrations are spontaneous flows made by individual Filipino nurses who rationally calculate professional earnings in both countries, and then migrate because the nursing salary in the United States is higher. This notion obscures the very important and complicated roles that both Philippine and U.S. governments, recruitment agencies, and professional nursing organizations, as well as the Filipino nurse migrants themselves, have played in facilitating this form of migration. Rendered invisible is the *culture of migration,* the ways in which narratives about the promise of immigration to the United States — narratives circulated by the media as well as Filipino nurse migrants already in the United States — shape Filipino nurses' desire to migrate abroad. Also rendered invisible are the ways U.S. hospital recruiters have collaborated across national boundaries with Philippine travel and recruitment agencies in their aggressive recruitment of Filipino nurses to work in their hospitals, collaborations that illuminate what Jon Goss and Bruce Lindquist have called the *institutionalization of migration.*[12] The lack of study about this culture and institutionalization of Filipino nurse migration to the United States, then, perpetuates a critical void. Little has been written about the exploitation faced by Filipino nurses from Philippine and American recruiters and their American hospital employers, the scapegoating of Filipino immigrants in the United States during difficult political times, and the absence of professional solidarity between Filipino and American nurses. All of these issues complicate and critique the popular narratives about the promise of American immigration.

The studies that include Filipino nurse migrants also marginalize and simplify the very complex and dynamic history of the colonial relationship between the United States and the Philippines. When the history of U.S. colonialism in the Philippines is mentioned, it is often in the context of an Americanized educational system that ambiguously predisposed Filipinos to American culture and customs. At stake here is the insidious persistence of the interrelated myths of U.S. exceptionalism and benevolence, which claim that Americans embraced their "little brown brothers" in the Philippines with what Vicente Rafael has called "white love."[13] According to these myths, America's tutelage of Filipinos bestowed on Filipinos the enlightened American systems of education, infrastructure, and public health, thus distinguishing Americans from their brutal Euro-

pean colonial counterparts. Rendered invisible are the ways U.S. colonialism in the Philippines created an Americanized training hospital system that eventually prepared Filipino women to work as nurses in the
United States as opposed to the Philippines. Furthermore, despite their
reformist intentions, American physicians and nurses in the Philippines
during the U.S. colonial period helped shape, as they were shaped by, a
culture of U.S. imperialism that created racialized hierarchies, with
Americans on top and Filipinos below.

Michael Salman and Matthew Jacobsen have astutely observed that
these pernicious myths of U.S. exceptionalism and benevolence persist in
more contemporary times through the erasure of the violent conquest of
the Philippines in Stanley Karnow's sentimental history of America's
empire in the Philippines and in David Grubin's profile of Theodore
Roosevelt for the PBS *American Presidents* series.[14] In addition, these
myths are refashioned and perpetuated today in U.S. immigration narratives popularized by the media, which claim that the United States continues to incorporate the "Third World" into its national borders to the
benefit of Asian, Latino, and African immigrants, but at the expense of
"Americans," a racialized identity most often portrayed as the industrious
white worker who supports immigrants through taxes, but then suffers
job losses and social services to these "foreigners."[15] While the campaigns
for California's Proposition 187 illustrated how working-class Mexican
immigrants served as the quintessential racialized and classed scapegoats
in this narrative, the highly educated and highly skilled backgrounds of
professional Asian immigrants have not made them immune to similar
anger and resentment, most recently demonstrated in the racialized per-
secution of nuclear physicist Wen Ho Lee.[16] Such anger and resentment are also directed toward foreign nurses and, by extension, Filipino
nurses. For example, in the late 1970s, when a U.S. nursing commission
proposed creating and financing an examination for foreign nurses before their migration to the United States, one American nurse responded
bitterly, "Scholarships and traineeships for *our own students* are always in
a precarious state . . . yet there are these thousands of dollars to spend on
having foreign-trained nurses immigrate."[17]

Such narratives erase the history of U.S. imperialism by suggesting
that Filipino nurse migrants exploit America (and not the other way
around); equally disturbing is the benevolent rhetoric used to describe
contemporary Filipino nurse migration as another, more recent "good"

outcome of U.S. colonialism in the Philippines. For example, at the 1998 roundtable on U.S. immigration history at the American Historical Association annual meeting, Rudolph Vecoli commented, "The Filipino nurses . . . who migrated to the United States surely enjoyed improved life opportunities because of the colonial history of the Philippines. Is it possible that some good could have come from imperialism?"[18] Although Filipino nurses did benefit from colonial nursing training in specific ways and at specific times, Vecoli's comments take the "good" that came out of colonialism out of its global and historical context, and simplify the complex and dynamic colonial relationship between the United States and the Philippines by romanticizing America's ability to provide opportunities for Filipino nurse migrants and erasing U.S. imperialism's, as well as the contemporary international labor market's, racialist and exploitive effects.

The major objectives of this book are to fill a gap in our knowledge about a unique and important form of contemporary professional migration to the United States and to challenge these myths of U.S. exceptionalism and benevolence through a transnational history of Filipino nurse migrations to the United States throughout the twentieth century. This book locates the formation of this racialized, gendered, and classed transnational labor force in the U.S. colonial presence in the Philippines; analyzes its development into a form of mass migration in the 1950s and 1960s; and critically explores how the experiences of recent Filipino nurse migrants have challenged some of the "promises" of American immigration: citizenship, opportunity, and equality. This book pays close attention to the voices and experiences of the Filipino nurses themselves and treats them as historical agents to contest the ways in which Filipino nurse migrants have been represented as commodified units of labor. It also highlights the multiple subjectivities involved in this migration — the views of American nurses and their professional nursing organizations; Philippine government and health officials; and American government officials and hospital employers — to show how nursing and migration in the twentieth century has meant different things (professional advancement, cheap labor, nation building, and national betrayal) to different individuals and collectivities on both sides of the ocean at specific moments in time.

I make four major arguments. First, the origins of Filipino nurse migration to the United States are not new, but rather, lie in early twentieth-century U.S. colonialism in the Philippines. Second, the desire of Filipino nurses to migrate abroad cannot be reduced to an economic logic, but rather reflects individual and collective desire for a unique form of social, cultural, and economic success obtainable only outside the national borders of the Philippines. Third, the culture of U.S. imperialism — specifically, its racialized social hierarchies — does not end with Philippine independence from the United States in 1946, but persists even in more recent times and continues to inform and shape the reception and incorporation of Filipino nurses in the United States. Fourth, although the development of a Filipino nurse migrant labor force has been shaped by ideologies of Philippine and U.S. nation building, Filipino nurse migrations to the United States need to be understood fundamentally as transnational processes, involving the flow of people, goods, services, images, and ideas across national boundaries.

Through its broad chronology, transnational emphasis, feminist analysis, and Philippine and Filipino American focus, this book engages with and hopes to expand and reconceptualize Asian American, migration, labor, and women's studies in multiple, interrelated ways. First, my emphasis on the imperial origins of contemporary migrations to the United States revises Asian American histories that have marginalized Asian professional migrations as a post-1965 phenomenon.[19] The liberalization of U.S. immigration policy codified in the 1965 Immigration Act does not explain why so many Filipinos, and specifically Filipino women, have become nurses. Broader questions are left unanswered: Why has the "developing" country of the Philippines emerged in the late twentieth century to provide professional nursing care for "developed" countries such as the United States? What enables and compels so many Filipino nurses to work abroad? Furthermore, although recent studies, most notably Amy Kaplan and Donald Pease's anthology *Cultures of United States Imperialism,* and Gilbert M. Joseph, Catherine C. Legrand, and Ricardo D. Salvatore's anthology *Close Encounters of Empire,* have brought more scholarly attention to the cultural dimensions of American imperialism, the intersections between American imperialism and U.S. immigration patterns have not been fully explored.[20] Sociologists such as Alejandro Portes and József Böröcz have importantly acknowledged the roles that conquest and colonization have played as precursors to labor migration patterns, yet they do not analyze the ways these themes endure in more contemporary times. Rather, they treat previous Western colonial penetration and its resulting migration flows as an earlier stage distinct from more contemporary "spontaneous labor flows," which they argue are primarily a result of worldwide cultural diffusion.[21] In the field of U.S. immigration history, the links between U.S. imperialism and immigration are barely acknowledged. As George Sánchez observed, "While the United States has clearly developed as an imperial power, and that imperialism (as well as previous colonial adventures) has directly and indirectly led to specific migrations to the United States, few American immigration historians have critically distinguished these forms of colonial migrations."[22]

Second, this study participates in the project outlined by Paul Ong, Edna Bonacich, and Lucie Cheng, who argue in their anthology on the new Asian immigration to Los Angeles that new immigration and labor trends, in particular the shift toward higher-educated, professional immigrants from Asia, need to be explained.[23] My study pushes the theoretical framework for this project further by taking seriously gender as a category of analysis. The ways in which race, nationality, gender, and class have shaped the experiences of Asian professional immigrant women have been virtually ignored in both ethnic and women's studies. The study of professional migrant women workers is often subsumed under the categories of highly educated laborers *or* migrant women workers in general. For example, although the Asian American and migration studies scholarship on Asian highly educated labor migration has included women, it has not paid close attention to gender as a useful category of analysis. In other words, this scholarship has tended to focus on the historical, economic, and demographic commonalties of all Asian professional migrant workers regardless of gender. And although the feminist scholarship on migrant women workers takes gender seriously in its analysis, the unique educational and socioeconomic backgrounds of professional migrant women workers are often lumped together with those of domestic workers and prostitutes.

The migration of Filipino nurses offers a unique lens through which to view the *intersections* of some of the most salient racialized, gendered, and classed dynamics of contemporary migration to the United States: the unintended exponential increase in immigration from Asia, the feminization of contemporary labor migration, and the significant percentage of highly skilled/professional immigrants. Although U.S. politicians did not expect the Immigration Act of 1965 to increase immigration from Asia, by the late 1980s the Philippines became the second largest sending country of immigrants to the United States, second only to Mexico.[24] Contemporary immigration patterns also reveal that women can no longer be marginalized in migration studies as wives, children, or other relatives that male migrants leave behind. In the United States, almost two-thirds of the 4.4 million documented immigrants between 1966 and 1978 were women.[25] Finally, between 1961 and 1972, approximately three hundred thousand scientific, technical, and professional workers from "developing" countries migrated to Western nations, primarily to Australia, Canada, and the United States. Asian countries played a significant role in this "brain flow," accounting for 72 percent of this type of migration to the United States.[26] Although these contemporary demographic shifts in the United States are often looked at separately, Filipino nurse migrants embody all three of these major changes.

Third, this book reconceptualizes the field of the history of nursing through its exploration of a new racialized and gendered professional labor force. In the historiography of American nursing, Darlene Clark Hine conceptualized the American nursing profession as an arena for racial conflict and cooperation in *Black Women in White*.[27] My work continues Hine's critique of the American nursing profession and, at the same time, provides a new international and transnational framework for this critique by analyzing factors such as national origin and citizenship as well as race. I re-present contemporary U.S. nursing as an *international* arena for the conflict and cooperation of predominantly women workers worldwide.

By continuing Hine's critique of American nursing as well as providing a new context for such a critique, I acknowledge the significance of race as a category of analysis in the history of nursing, but I also resist the way a U.S. black-and-white dichotomy has dominated American analyses of race. By conceptualizing a new international and transnational framework from which to view the nursing profession, I argue that the significance of a history that takes into account the experiences of Filipino nurses in the United States is qualitative and not simply quantitative (i.e., including another "minority" group in the picture of American nursing for more equitable representation). Indeed, taking into account the experiences of Filipino nurses in the United States changes that picture. For example, in the early twentieth century, while white American nurses excluded African American nurses from their training hospitals and professional organizations in the United States, they also established nursing training schools in the Philippines and actively recruited young Filipino girls to train under their supervision. This benevolent treatment of Filipino nurses was no less racist in the contexts of American colonialism, manifest destiny, and the white (wo)man's burden. However, in the early twentieth century, race and nursing functioned quite differently — on social, cultural, political, and institutional levels — for African American and Filipino nurses.

Finally, given my emphasis on international and transnational contexts, this book engages with the concerns raised by American studies and Asian American studies scholars in the past decade about the U.S.-centric nature of these fields. American studies scholars have questioned the limitations of the study of American experiences within the United States and have expressed the need to critically analyze the paradigms and assumptions of U.S. nationalist thinking, a move that Barbara Brinson Curiel, David Kazanjian, Katherine Kinney, Steven Mailloux, Jay Mechling, John Carlos Rowe, George Sánchez, Shelly Streeby, and Henry Yu have termed "post-nationalist American studies."[28] Similar concerns have emerged in the field of Asian American studies, where conferences and symposia at Harvard University, University of Washington, and California State University have focused on re-"visioning" Asian American studies. Until very recently, Asian American studies scholarship has privileged the experiences of Asian Americans within a U.S. nation–bound context and has expressed ambivalence about Asian Americans' transnational linkages to Asia.[29] Scholars have done this in part to make the important point that Asian Americans have lived in the United States for over 150 years, yet contemporary demographics have compelled Asian American studies scholars to rethink their methodological approaches.

Contemporary Asian migration to the United States has shaped a very different, diverse, and complex Asian America. In the late twentieth century, Asian America has grown considerably from the influx of immigrants and refugees from Southeast and South Asia. By the late 1980s, the Philippines, Vietnam, and India were among the top ten sending nations of immigrants to the United States. A majority of the contemporary Asian American population is foreign-born. New Asian American communities have been established on the West Coast and in New York, Massachusetts, Illinois, Minnesota, Texas, Virginia, and Georgia.

These recent dramatic demographic shifts, combined with the accessibility of new technologies such as international air travel and electronic mail, have brought heightened awareness to the transnational dimensions of new American immigrants' lives. However, transnational frameworks are also useful for an understanding of earlier periods of migration. For example, Madeline Hsu's study of transnationalism and migration between the United States and South China focuses on the period from 1882 to 1943. For Hsu, the late nineteenth- and early twentieth-century migration patterns of Taishanese Americans highlight the need to study migration beyond the borders of nation-states and through the contexts of transnational and global processes.[30] Similarly, I argue that, although contemporary demographics and technologies raise more awareness about the need for new frameworks of analysis that go beyond national boundaries, the transnational context for Filipino nurse migration to the United States emerges in the early 1900s, and not after World War II or 1965.

This book is organized chronologically and thematically in three parts. Part I, "Nurturing Empire," explores the ways ideologies of gender intersected with those of race and class and shaped and informed U.S. colonial practices and agendas, in particular its medical practices and agendas. Chapter 1 examines the introduction of nursing in the Philippines during U.S. colonial rule from the multiple perspectives of American and Filipino nurses. Chapter 2 analyzes the ways in which the creation of an Americanized training hospital system in the Philippines established several preconditions that enabled Filipino nurse mass migration abroad in the late twentieth century.

Part II, "Caring Unbound," focuses on the development of Filipino nurse migration into a form of mass migration to the United States after World War II and the often contradictory motivations, agendas, and outcomes that accompanied it. In Chapter 3 I explore the complexities of the U.S. Exchange Visitor Program of the 1950s and 1960s, a program rooted in cold war politics, which inadvertently facilitated the first wave of Filipino nurse mass migration to the United States. In Chapter 4 I analyze contemporary government policies in both the United States and the Philippines — specifically, the U.S. Immigration Act of 1965 and the Philippine government's institutionalization of labor export in the early 1970s — that furthered the mass migration of Filipino nurses abroad and to the United States in particular.

Part III, "Still the Golden Door?," challenges celebratory narratives about professional migrants' international mobility and the promises of American immigration through an examination of the scapegoating of two Filipino immigrant nurses, Filipina Narciso and Leonora Perez, and the exploitation of Filipino nurses with temporary work visas, also known as H-1 visas. Chapter 5 compares two mass-murder cases in the United States involving Filipino nurses: the 1966 Richard Speck massacre, in which two of Speck's victims and the only survivor of the massacre were Filipino exchange nurses, and the 1975 Veterans Administration Hospital murders in Ann Arbor, Michigan, in which Filipino immigrant nurses Narciso and Perez were convicted, though later acquitted, of poisoning and conspiracy. I illustrate how the representations of Filipino nurses in these cases reflected the dynamic stereotypes of Filipino nurses, stereotypes steeped in a culture of U.S. imperialism. Chapter 6 traces the development of Filipino nurse organizations in the United States in the late 1970s, organizations that formed partly as a response to the exploitation and discrimination faced by Filipino nurses with temporary work visas. I conclude with a brief discussion about more recent controversies surrounding Filipino nurses in the United States regarding illegal migration and English-only policies and the ways in which contemporary U.S. migration patterns, specifically its recruitment of Filipino nurses, illustrate how much the United States has become similar to, as opposed to distinct from, other developed countries.

I am intellectually indebted to the pioneering work of Asian American historians such as Sucheng Chan, Gary Okihiro, and Ronald Takaki, who have persuasively argued that the histories of Asian Americans matter, not only to Asian Americans, but to all students of American experiences. Yet I have been distressed by the scarcity of scholarly production in Filipino American history and the ways Chinese and Japanese American historical experiences have become almost synonymous with Asian American history.[31] As Sucheng Chan concluded in her essay on Asian American historiography, "Despite the steady progress in Asian American historical scholarship, significant gaps remain. The most glaring is the absence of book-length studies on Filipino Americans."[32] As I write this introduction from my office at the University of Minnesota, Twin

Cities, and reflect on my research and writing here during the past three years, the need for more scholarly work on Filipino American history has become painfully apparent to me. In terms of Filipino American history, one may not think of the state of Minnesota, with its comparatively small Filipino population as well as the West Coast–centric nature of Asian American studies scholarship. But recent events in this state reflect what Matthew Jacobsen has called the "modern art of forgetting": Americans' erasure of their imperial history.[33]

Minnesota's most recent claim to national fame has been its election of the "refreshing" Independent Party governor, former professional wrestler and commentator Jesse "The Body" Ventura. In his best-selling autobiography, *I Ain't Got Time to Bleed,* Ventura waxed nostalgic about his good old days as a Navy Seal stationed in the Philippines: "I loved the Philippines. I was stationed at Subic, and I loved going into Olongapo. It was more like the Wild West than any other place on earth. In Olongapo, there's a one-mile stretch of road that has 350 bars and 10,000 girls on it every night. . . . To the kid I was then, it was paradise. . . . When a girl went with you in Olongapo, there was no question about what you were going to do. In the States, you had to wine 'em and dine 'em. At that point in my life, I was barely out of my teens; I wasn't into wining and dining. The libido was still in charge. A lot of my buddies felt that way too."[34]

As I have argued elsewhere, what is important about Ventura's representation of the Philippines is what it excludes as well as includes.[35] The use of Filipino women to embody a feminized Philippine "paradise" for the heterosexual desires of American men is a central part of this depiction. The rhetoric of "love" elides the history of a violent U.S. dominance in the archipelago. Invisible are the colonial and neocolonial relationships of inequality between the United States and the Philippines, and more specifically the history of U.S. military presence in the islands and its legacies of prostitution, disease, and environmental destruction. Also invisible are the migrations of Filipinos to the United States that have been shaped by this U.S. military presence in the Philippines, such as the active recruitment of Filipino men into the U.S. Navy, which, by 1970, contributed to a larger number of Filipinos in the U.S. Navy (fourteen thousand) than in the entire Philippine Navy.[36]

More recently, the Philippine Study Group of Minnesota spearheaded a campaign to install a correction to a historically inaccurate plaque in the

Rotunda of the Capitol Building in St. Paul, which commemorated the service of Minnesota volunteers in the Philippines during the Spanish-American War. According to the original plaque, these Minnesotans "battled to free the oppressed peoples of the Philippine Islands, who suffered under the despotic rule of Spain." The Philippine Study Group together with other Filipino American organizations successfully convinced the Minnesota legislature to correct the text of the plaque to acknowledge that the Spanish-American War "was fought to defeat Spain, not to free the Filipinos" and that, soon after Spain's surrender to the United States in 1898, Filipinos fought unsuccessfully for full independence against the United States in the Philippine-American War.[37] Although the plaque correction is a victory in this particular struggle, legacies of empire and war continue to haunt Filipino Americans, most notably Filipino American war veterans who served under the U.S. Armed Forces of the Far East during World War II but continue to struggle for their veterans' benefits. These examples of America's "forgetfulness" become especially important in light of the powerful impact they have on the lived experiences of Filipinos and Filipino Americans.

Thus, it is my hope that this book contributes to shaping the contours of a Filipino American history, a history that is unafraid to cross national as well as disciplinary boundaries; that rigorously critiques the exploitive and enduring legacies of U.S. imperialism and colonialism in the contemporary lives of Filipinos and Filipino Americans; and that sustains, but also moves beyond, a critique of Filipino Americans as "forgotten" Asian Americans through the analytical study of those cultural terrains where Filipinos have made an impact on American society and global history. By focusing on the imperial origins of Filipino nurse migrations to the United States and their connection to the more recent experiences of the Filipino nurse migrants themselves, this book is one step in this direction.

PART I

Nurturing Empire

Nursing in the Philippines has a history on which we may look back
with satisfaction, for, while carried on almost entirely by Americans in
the early days of the occupation, its speedy adoption into the life and
education of the Filipinos themselves and its wonderfully rapid
development have probably not been surpassed elsewhere.
— LAVINIA DOCK, Secretary of the International Council of
Nursing, *A History of Nursing,* 1912

A modern hospital has been constructed even in the heart of the wild
man's country, and through the ministrations of the doctor and the
nurse, as well as a teacher, and other influences, these people are being
brought rapidly from head-hunting savages to useful and productive
people. — DR. M. D. KNEEDLER, Medical Director of the Insular Life
Insurance Company in the Philippines, letter to President Woodrow
Wilson, 1913

Yes, to see America and have the opportunity to further my studies has
been my dream ever since I learned of the great country. . . . I made up
my mind to take up nursing against the objection of my father.
— PATROCINIO MONTELLANO, writing about her student
nurse experiences in the late 1910s, "Years That Count," 1962

CHAPTER I

Nursing Matters

Women and U.S. Colonialism in the Philippines

As she reflected on her 1920s sojourn to the United States, Filipino nurse Patrocinio Montellano reminisced fondly about her experiences in "the Land of Promise."[1] During her four-year stay, she traveled throughout the United States working as a nurse in Honolulu and New York City, and furthered her nursing education by taking postgraduate courses in San Francisco, Cleveland, and Washington, D.C. Montellano secured her employment through American individuals such as William Musgrave, a former director of Philippine General Hospital, and funded her postgraduate studies through scholarships she had earned with recommendations from Mary Cole, director of the Southwestern Division of the American Red Cross. Upon Montellano's return to the Philippines in 1924, she became field representative and nurse supervisor of the Philippine Chapter of the American Red Cross.

Montellano's experiences of education, work, and travel would not have been possible only a few decades earlier, when the Philippines was still under Spanish colonial rule. Before the U.S. annexation of the Philippines at the turn of the twentieth century, Spain's colonial educational system offered distinct and unequal opportunities for Filipinos based on gender. Only limited numbers of Filipino girls received some primary education in Spanish charitable institutions. The Spanish university in the Philippines, University of Santo Tomas, excluded women from obtaining higher education until a School of Midwifery was founded in 1879.[2]

In the context of specialized health care work, midwifery was the only area open to Filipino women during Spanish colonial rule. Filipino women cared for sick family members and friends at home, and Filipinos also consulted indigenous healers. However, in Spanish colonial hospitals and other medical institutions, primarily Spanish friars and priests cared for the sick. In 1862, Sisters of Charity and a European nurse arrived to work at San Juan de Dios Hospital. Additionally, Spanish surgeons, or *practicantes,* and the Filipino male physicians who had graduated from the University of Santo Tomas's School of Medicine practiced general as well as specialized areas of medicine. Furthermore, in the late nineteenth century, the Spanish colonial government encouraged elite Filipino men, known as *ilustrados,* to further their education abroad in European universities such as University of Barcelona and Central University of Madrid.[3] The most famous ilustrado, Philippine national hero Jose Rizal, was a doctor of medicine. Such opportunities were unavailable to Filipino women. Given these historical contexts, it is no wonder that Montellano characterized the United States as a "land of promise."

Although some scholars have suggested that American colonialism's effect on Filipino women was marginal, Montellano's story reveals some of the watershed changes during the U.S. colonial period in the Philippines that impacted young Filipino women.[4] These changes included the introduction of new professions, such as nursing, and educational and travel opportunities in the United States. From the beginning of U.S. colonial rule, the introduction of these new forms of labor and opportunities abroad were closely linked. Montellano's story further illustrates that, soon after U.S. annexation of the Philippines, important transnational ties had already developed between Americans and Filipino women. These ties enabled Montellano's socioeconomic as well as geographic mobility. American physicians and nurses helped her to secure employment and educational opportunities in the United States. This experience abroad in turn helped her earn an advanced nursing position on her return to the Philippines. Although Americans undoubtedly played a significant role in promoting these opportunities for Filipino women, Montellano's memories also reveal that her determination and desire to study nursing and to see America — even against the objection of her father, who thought that she was "small and frail and too young" — was also a crucial element in the implementation of U.S. colonial projects.[5]

This chapter examines the introduction of nursing in the Philippines during the early U.S. colonial period from the multiple perspectives of American and Filipino nurses. These perspectives highlight the complex ways in which ideologies of gender intersected with those of race and class and shaped U.S. colonial agendas and practices. While the volu-

minous literature on women and imperialism has made important interventions that challenge the "masculine" nature of imperialism, the scant
attention paid to American women's participation in U.S. colonialism in
the Philippines continues to erase America's imperial past in general, and
perpetuates the popular amnesia about U.S. colonialism in the archipelago in particular.[6] Like the recent scholarly work by Louise Michele
Newman, Vicente Rafael, and Laura Wexler on white American women's
participation in American imperialism, which has contested this erasure,
I argue that U.S. colonial nursing in the Philippines played a critical role
in the formation of American modernity, specifically in American wom-
en's construction of themselves as civilized women.[7] However, unlike
this scholarship that has focused primarily on white American women's
narratives and subjectivity, this chapter highlights the impact of colonial
nursing on Filipino women's identities and desires.

The perspectives of Filipino nurses merit close attention because they
reveal that the beliefs and actions of Filipinos as well as Americans were
integral to the establishment of Philippine nursing. They also illustrate
the complex ways that nursing and medicine in general provided professional opportunities for an elite group of Filipino women while simultaneously serving to legitimate U.S. colonial agendas that created as well as
confirmed racialized and gendered social hierarchies. Unlike other economic, political, and educational agendas in the colony, the popular
conceptualization of Western medicine as a universal humanitarian effort
to save lives continues to make it difficult for scholars and others to
critique its racialist and exploitive effects. As Reynaldo Ileto noted,
"Even nationalist writers in the Philippines find it impossible to interro-
gate the established notion that among the blessings of American colonial rule was a sanitary regime which saved countless Filipino lives."[8]
However, scholarship in the growing field of science, medicine, and
imperialism has effectively revised heroic portrayals of Western medical
practices in colonized areas by arguing that these practices served as
instruments of colonial subjugation and control.[9] Yet many of these
studies focus on large-scale sanitation projects and diseases, often render-
ing colonized peoples as coerced and unfortunate victims. I argue that
the U.S. introduction of professional nursing greatly influenced Filipino
women in ways that were both liberating and exploitative. Although the
introduction of professional nursing in the Philippines presented new
opportunities for Filipino women, it needs to be understood as part of a

larger U.S. colonial agenda that racialized Filipinos and Americans under the guise of benevolent reform. Furthermore, although Philippine nursing was shaped by both Filipinos and Americans, the study and practice of nursing took place in the context of unequal colonial relationships.

Finally, this chapter documents a period of transnational mobility that has been marginalized in Filipino American history. In the early twentieth century, American and Filipino nurses shaped Philippine nursing through travel as well as teaching, training, and practice. American nurses traveled to the Philippines to teach and practice nursing during the early part of the U.S. colonial period, and eventually returned to the United States. As Montellano's story illustrates, Filipino nurses also traveled to the United States to study and practice nursing and then returned to the Philippines. This multidirectional mobility has been ignored in Asian American histories that foreground Filipino migrations eastward to the United States, but have focused on Filipino male migrants, many of whom worked as migrant agricultural laborers and settled permanently in the United States.[10] Although these studies have importantly analyzed the racism and exploitation encountered by these Filipino men in America, more attention to other gendered forms of mobility during this period brings to light the transnational formation of new female labor regimes, such as nursing, during the U.S. colonial period. The formation of this gendered labor force would lay the foundation for the significant migrations of Filipino nurses later in the twentieth century.

THE RACE FOR EMPIRE

The introduction of nursing in the Philippines was part of a larger U.S. colonial and medical agenda that racialized Filipinos and Americans in the context of reform. Health care personnel contributed to the overall U.S. colonial project of preparing Filipinos for self-rule through the introduction of American medical practices. American medicine, they believed, would transform Filipino bodies into a people capable of self-government. "Filipino health" became a forceful metaphor for the primary objectives of U.S. colonialism. As Victor Heiser, director of health in the Philippine Islands, claimed, "To summarize, it is to be understood that the health of these people is the vital question of the Islands. To transform them from the weak and feeble race we have found them into the strong, healthy, and enduring people that they yet may become is to lay the foundations for the successful future of the country."[11] Such concerns for the welfare of Filipinos complemented America's "benevolent assimilation" of the Philippines, which, as U.S. President William McKinley proclaimed in 1898, brought Americans to the Philippines "not as invaders or conquerors, but as friends."[12]

However, these reformist intentions depended on the social and scientific construction of Filipino bodies as weak, diseased, and therefore racially inferior. In turn, American bodies also needed to be reinvented as vigorous, healthy, and therefore racially superior. U.S. health care personnel popularized these constructions of Filipino and American bodies in letters, reports, articles, and books that legitimized and rationalized such racism through medicine. For example, in Victor Heiser's 1910 article on "unsolved health problems peculiar to the Philippines," he presented Filipinos as a primitive people helplessly lost in a timeless past with little hope of entering modernity if not for the tutelage — and specifically the medical tutelage — of modern Americans: "We are practically cleaning up these Islands, left foul and insanitary and diseased by generations of hygienically ignorant peoples. We are stamping out the conflagration of disease started long before American occupation, and not until it is stamped out can we look forward to the modern problems which come so temptingly before us. . . . We are draining the land, as it were, before beginning the constructive health projects which are going to make these people the strong and healthy race we intend them to be."[13]

Although America's "benevolent" colonialism has contributed to the popular ideology of American exceptionalism, which claims that the United States has a national character distinct from other colonial powers, American colonialism was not wholly unique in its view and application of Western medicine in the Philippines. General similarities can be drawn between American and European colonial medicine. For example, American imperialism in the Philippines, like nineteenth- and early twentieth-century British imperialism in India and South Africa, utilized Western medicine to justify the "white man's burden" overseas, to create racialized hierarchies of peoples, and to dominate those who differed from them culturally and physically. By extension, American nursing in the Philippines functioned in similar ways.

In recent histories of European and American imperialism, Western medicine's "power to heal" and colonizers' justifications for domination over the colonized are inextricably linked. Metaphors of healing in eighteenth-century British poetry and travel accounts provided ideological justification for Britain's nineteenth- and early twentieth-century "humane imperialism" in the "suffering abandon" of South Africa.[14] Similarly, "suffering" among Filipinos justified American colonial medical intervention in the Philippines. After American victories over cholera in the United States in the 1830s and 1850s, an outbreak of cholera in the Philippines in the early 1900s gave American military surgeons and sanitation personnel a righteous purpose in their surveillance of the islands.[15]

Western medicine functioned in different areas of the world to penetrate the colonized's bodies through statistical and laboratory studies. Medical personnel then used these studies to authenticate cultural and racial hierarchies. In the 1840s, British studies of malaria conducted in India involved spleen examinations of approximately twelve thousand Indian villagers. In the early 1900s, American scientists in government laboratories in the Philippines conducted studies of Igorots' stools to study parasites. These laboratory studies linked native bodies to dirt and disease. In the late nineteenth century, British medical officers claimed that the bodies of Indian camp servants, prostitutes, and food vendors "carried" enteric fever into the presence of British soldiers.[16] Similarly, Heiser associated Filipino bodies with disease, describing them as "incubators of leprosy."[17]

In British and American colonies, the colonized often resisted such Western medical intervention when it opposed their own social beliefs and practices. In nineteenth-century India, the vast majority of Indians refused British vaccination to prevent smallpox, opting instead for their traditional ways of surviving the epidemic, such as religious rituals and variolation.[18] In the early twentieth-century Philippines, Filipino cholera victims refused to take American anticholera drugs and continued to consult indigenous healers, such as *curanderos*. Steeped in their belief in their power to heal, British and American medical personnel linked the colonized's social practices to ignorance and societal backwardness. One British medical officer criticized Hindus as "stupid and insensible" because they refused smallpox vaccination.[19] Paralleling such conclusions, an American chief quarantine officer contrasted Filipinos who opposed American anticholera measures such as quarantine with "intelligent Americans or Europeans."[20]

The introduction of nursing in the Philippines differed from previous American medical interventions because it involved the agitation and participation of American women in the Philippines. Although Edward Carter, a U.S. Army surgeon and Philippine Commissioner of Health, had recommended the establishment of a training school for Filipino nurses before the Philippine Commission as early as 1903, and although the Baptist Foreign Mission Society had established the Iloilo Mission Hospital School of Nursing in 1906, it was not until 1907, with the urging of Mary Coleman, dean of women at the Philippine Normal School, that the U.S. colonial government established a nursing school.[21] Nursing education, like teaching and missionary work, in the Philippines provided white American women with a sense of purpose in the colony. Similar to British nurses in colonial West Africa, nursing offered white American women an international avenue for heroism, one still dominated by, though no longer entirely in the hands of, male medical personnel.[22] Yet, although white American women as opposed to men were predominantly in charge of the training of Filipino nurses, and although they probably conceived their nursing duties as a humane and progressive alternative to traditionally masculine forms of imperial violence, nursing education "nurtured empire" as it reinforced many of the racialist functions and beliefs of Western medicine.[23] The multivolume history of nursing and its section on the Philippines written by Lavinia Dock in 1912 offers one prominent American nurse's interpretation of colonial nursing in the archipelago.

Lavinia Dock was an activist in the professionalization of U.S. nursing and the internationalization of professional nursing. She served as the first secretary of the American Society of Superintendents of Training Schools in the United States and Canada (later known as the National League of Nursing Education) and helped to found the Nurses' Associated Alumnae of the United States and Canada (later known as the American Nurses Association), organizations at the forefront of professionalizing American nursing. In addition, Dock served as the first secretary of the International Council of Nursing from 1900 to 1922. With Isabel Stewart, she coauthored the first history of nursing that covered the development of nursing from ancient times until her day and included its development in other countries as well as the United States. Dock also wrote the first pharmacology textbook for nurses, supported the founding of the *American Journal of Nursing* in 1900, and served as one of its editors until 1923. A passionate advocate for social reforms of the Progressive Era and woman's suffrage and a self-proclaimed pacifist with "a strong sympathy with oppressed classes, a lively sense of justice and a keen love of what we mean by 'freedom' and 'liberty,'" Dock supported American medical agendas in the Philippines in the name of a humane imperialism.[24]

Yet, like other American white women writing about the Philippine colony in the early twentieth century, Dock's writing disavowed violent U.S. imperial agendas.[25] She excluded discussion on the various, and sometimes violent, ways that Filipinos resisted U.S. medical practices. Some Filipinos killed U.S. inspectors who conducted the cholera search and surveillance missions. Filipino cholera victims physically resisted taking anticholera drugs, so that American doctors at times had to use force when administering their medicine.[26] Despite these violent forms of American imposition and Filipino resistance, for Dock, the continued presence of disease in the Philippines justified the need for more American medical intervention in the form of nursing: "With an infant mortality rate of forty-four percent (of total number of deaths), there is an immense field right here for visiting nurses' settlements."[27]

Dock's international vision of nursing in the Philippines complemented U.S. colonial agendas by echoing imperial narratives that justified U.S. colonialism in the Philippines on the basis of Filipinos' poor health. As she explained, "To establish the Filipino people physically is to insure their future effectiveness and prosperity. It should be the basis of all the educational work of the islands. To decrease the high infant mortality, to stamp out small-pox, cholera, tuberculosis, malaria, hookworm, beri-beri, and many other diseases which are retarding the progress of the Filipinos is absolutely necessary in order to build scientific and industrial education on a substantial foundation."[28]

The "physical establishment" of Filipinos involved both theoretical and practical forms of Western medical knowledge. U.S. medical personnel accepted the model of diseases and their spread through germ theory, the late nineteenth-century development in European medicine that claimed that microorganisms were the cause of specific diseases. Practically, they aimed to control the spread of germs through specific sanitary and hygienic measures, such as daily washing, sterilization, and quarantine. In her writing, Dock reified the beliefs of other U.S. medical personnel that such knowledge was elusive to Filipinos because of their indigenous social practices. According to Dock, young Filipino women who were targeted to train as nurses suffered from the lack of "rudimentary knowledge" about sanitation as a result of the prevailing Filipino "primitive customs." As she claimed with a hint of exasperation about the opening of the first government nursing school in the Philippines in 1907, "The idea of women nursing was an entirely foreign one to the Filipino people. To them the work seemed menial and wholly beneath a person of any family or birth. Not only did this idea have to be entirely overcome with both parents and young women, but the latter, as students, had to be grounded in the very A-B-C of hygiene and sanitation — rudimentary knowledge which, in our country, is assimilated we know not when or how — it is almost inborn. It is difficult for us to realise that some of the most primitive customs prevail among persons of more or less education in the Philippines. All this was uphill work, but the school was finally started."[29]

The training of Filipino nurses, like America's medical mission against the cholera epidemic, involved the imposition of control over Filipinos' social beliefs and practices regarding class and gender. As Dock herself admitted, the notion of Filipino women working as nurses was an idea that had to be "entirely overcome" both by Filipinos in general and elite Filipinos in particular. Their strong objections were probably related to the training of Filipino nurses in hospitals, which had become the sites for the training of student nurses in the late nineteenth-century United States. Elite Filipinos regarded the Spanish colonial hospitals as places where those who were so unfortunate as not to have homes would spend their last days until death. Furthermore, during the cholera epidemic, rumors spread among Filipinos that Americans poisoned cholera victims upon their arrival at the hospitals.[30]

The training of Filipino nurses involved not only spatial control within the hospital workplace; it also involved corporeal control in terms of clothing. Elite Filipino families, from which Americans originally recruited potential nursing students, opposed the use of the American-style nursing uniform, as its absence of a long train signified lower-class status. Echoing imperial narratives that cast all Filipinos in a timeless past and ignored Filipino cultural differences, Dock referred to an essential "Filipino costume" and characterized the donning of the nursing uniform by Filipinos as yet "another struggle": "The Filipino has worn the same style of costume for about three hundred years. This dress has a long train which carries with it class distinction. It is almost symbolical of the leisure or wealthy upper class: the longer the train, the higher the class, absence of train, lack of class. To abolish this costume even for the period of 'duty,' was therefore, something to accomplish, but it was done, and the student nurses now look most attractive in their striped, gingham uniforms, with white caps and aprons."[31]

Furthermore, the idea that Filipino *women* engaged in nursing was a gendered construction about the labor of nursing, which American nursing leaders in the Philippines actively had to reproduce in the archipelago. In the United States, while the nature of nursing as labor changed from being a last option for women in the mid–nineteenth century into more respectable and proper work for women by the early twentieth century, nursing was consistently "women's" work. Furthermore, sex segregation, in the form of a separate "women's sphere" that encompassed professional opportunities, was an integral part of the evolutionary logic of late nineteenth- and early twentieth-century white American women's "civilization" work. As Louise Newman points out in her generative work on the racial origins of feminism in the United States, "Evolutionist theories linked sexual differences with racial progress. 'Civilized' races were differentiated from 'primitive' races according to the specific sexual traits and gender roles that characterized the white middle classes. . . . the more civilized the race, the more the men and women of that race had to differ from one another."[32] Thus, Dock and other American nurses viewed Filipino women's nursing training as a foundational point from which to begin the uplift of the Filipino race. Her history of the establishment of Americanized nursing in the Philippines reveals that the American effort to impose American nursing customs involved the deliberate attempt to separate and exclude men from the labor of nursing: "When Miss McCalmont took charge of the nursing force in the Philippines, a peculiar state of affairs existed. All male patients, even the Americans, were cared for by male attendants only. In the men's wards, the nurses did only desk work, charting, and giving out medicines. Baths, treatments, and nearly all surgical dressings were done by the attendants, who were generally ex-army corps men, with even less than the ordinary training. . . . It seemed impossible to get the nurses back into the hospital habits of the United States, and an attempt was made to solve the problem by a training school for men."[33]

Finally, American colonial medicine and nursing enabled American medical personnel to biologically and socially reinvent American bodies and social practices. In the early 1900s, the American colonial government had established laboratories to study Filipino and American bodies in the archipelago. These laboratory studies, which included the disease surveys of parasites in Igorots' stools, for example, "re"-discovered Filipino bodies as a potentially dangerous type, a carrier of germs, parasites, and pathogens. Dock, again confirming the beliefs of other medical personnel, was probably referring to such laboratory studies when she claimed that "*investigation* has shown the impaired health and weakened condition of the Filipino people (who are not a strong or enduring race) to be largely due to the prevalence not only of tuberculosis, but of the hook-worm disease, which seems to have no equal in its capacity to enervate and undermine the system."[34] However, colonial laboratory studies also "re"-discovered American bodies as a resilient racial type. Focusing on the control of external factors, such as clothing or contact with the "natives," these studies concluded that American bodies could survive the tropical climate, once thought to be the source of the "white man's grave."[35]

Dock's history of nursing and the reproduction of late nineteenth-century American nursing reforms in the Philippines similarly invented a sanitized image of the United States. While Dock's insistence that Filipino young women "had to be grounded in the very A-B-C of hygiene and sanitation" revealed the very Westerncentric perspective from which notions of hygiene and sanitation were constructed and taught, her history also concealed the historical changes regarding hygiene and sanitation in the United States. Dock claimed that the "A-B-C of hygiene and sanitation" was "rudimentary knowledge which, in our country, is assimilated we know not when or how — it is almost inborn," suggesting that such knowledge among Americans was innate, biological, and immutable. However, before 1873, when the first training schools for nurses were opened in the United States, the hospital was an institution for society's marginal people, such as the poor. Dirt, vermin, and rampant cross-infection known as hospitalism were common.[36] Until the creation of the modern U.S. hospital after the Civil War, American patients in the nineteenth century, like Filipinos, tried to avoid hospitalization. It was not until the 1900s, when Lavinia Dock published her history of nursing, that nurses in American hospitals concentrated their efforts on incessant cleaning to promote what Dock referred to ahistorically as the "A-B-C of hygiene and sanitation."

CONFLICTS IN THE COLONY

Although colonial narratives by Victor Heiser and Lavinia Dock portrayed the objectives and accomplishments of U.S. colonial medicine and nursing as a unified and successful agenda, the lived experiences of American nurses in the Philippines fracture the seamlessness of such narratives. Their experiences reveal the frustrations and troubling outcomes of colonialism for the colonizers as well as the colonized and bring to light the struggles that U.S. colonial officials faced from American nurses, and not solely from Filipinos, which Dock's narrative led readers to believe. For example, Dock's heroic history of nursing in the Philippines masked the desperate struggles of U.S. officials to recruit American nurses to work in the colony. Throughout the early 1900s, the Philippine Civil Service Board sent letters to the U.S. Civil Service Commission and the Bureau of Insular Affairs that related the "considerable difficulty" in recruiting and retaining American nurses to work in the Philippine Civil Hospital (later known as Philippine General Hospital).[37]

The preferences of American medical and nursing supervisors in the Philippines contributed to this difficulty. In the early 1900s, W. S. Washburn, chairman of the Philippine Civil Service Board in Manila, noted that the Civil Hospital's attending physician and surgeon had objected to some of the previous nurse appointees from the United States. The physician had insisted that all of the nurse recruits had to have graduated from "recognized training schools" of not less than one hundred–bed hospitals. They needed to have at least one year's experience thereafter in general hospital work, and should not be over thirty-five years of age.[38]

U.S. colonial officials attempted to attract these American nurses to the Philippines through personal contacts at (what they considered to be) suitable U.S. nursing programs, such as those at Presbyterian Hospital in New York and Waltham Training School in Massachusetts. They requested that recruitment advertisements be placed in the *American Journal of Nursing*. They also scouted for potential recruits among American nurses who had taken examinations for the Panama and Indian Services, illustrating one way that nursing linked U.S. imperial agendas among peoples abroad as well as among American Indians domestically.

The U.S. Civil Service Commission allayed American nurses' concerns about their living conditions in the Philippines by publicizing the availability of modern hospital facilities and accommodations there. Such facilities helped to consolidate an Americanized "order out of the chaos" of the Philippine tropics.[39] If, as Vicente Rafael has observed in the writing of white American women in the colony, "imperialism appears as domesticity on the move," then nursing as a professional extension of U.S. domesticity could also be mobile in the form of modern hospital facilities built in the colony.[40] The U.S. Civil Service Commission described these facilities in this way: "Connected with the Philippine General Hospital there is a nurses' home built of reenforced concrete. This building is also new and has only been occupied since April last. It has all modern conveniences, including electric lights and fans, hot and cold water, large commodious verandas, and special provisions for out-door sleeping. New hospitals are in course of construction at a number of other places, and at all of the institutions where nurses are on duty they have modern accommodations."[41]

U.S. colonial officials also characterized nursing service in the Philippines as an exotic travel adventure. In her recruitment letter, Supervising Nurse of the Bureau of Health in the Philippines Mabel McCalmont highlighted that nursing service in the Philippines presented "an opportunity for travel so exceptional." She described the global adventures awaiting American nurses, emphasizing that the world could be consumed visually and experientially by modern women like themselves through nursing work in the colony: "In the first place, the fascinating trip by liner across the Pacific with the interesting stops of Honolulu, Hawaii; Yokohama, Kobe and Nagasaki, Japan; and Shanghai and Hongkong, China gives to the wide awake woman a glimpse into Oriental life, manners and customs, indelibly impressive and broadening. After termination of service here, the ambitious ones return via Europe, thus completing the circle of the globe and gaining an experience which is the desire of many, but which comes to but few."[42] Such writing helped to constitute a U.S. imperial gaze that presented the availability of "the rest of the world" to American nursing recruits to the Philippine colony.[43]

Despite these efforts, recruitment continued to be a struggle. American nurses acted on their own preferences regarding working conditions and, in doing so, also contributed to the difficulty of recruitment. They rejected service in the Philippines for various reasons. One nurse did not want to have an operating room assignment; another preferred to wait for a nurse opening in Panama; another refused to work with smallpox.[44]

Conflicts among U.S. nurses already working in the Philippines posed an even greater struggle. In the early 1910s, letters from Mabel McCalmont and Victor Heiser revealed that internal feuding between American nurses and their supervisors in the Civil Hospital disrupted the efficiency of nursing service and severely damaged the morale of those involved. Reports of theft of government property by American nurses and charges of emotional instability further complicated the situation.[45] Mabel McCalmont, who, in addition to her role as supervising nurse of the Bureau of Health also served as superintendent of the Civil Hospital, characterized the nursing situation at the Bureau and the hospital as "deplorable" and in an "almost hopeless condition" before she occupied her dual roles: "Discontent and insubordination were rife, loyalty was an unknown quantity, incompetent persons were at the helms, and the most wanton extravagance prevailed. This condition, tho' recognized, could not be remedied because of the lack of loyal and competent employees."[46]

While nursing supervisors blamed nurses for the disloyalty and inefficiency at the Bureau of Health, letters from American nurses presented another view that criticized the Philippine Civil Service for low salaries and accused their supervisors of inattentive leadership and unfair assignments. In 1913, nurses Alice Bruton and Mary Dugan wrote to Chief of the Bureau of Insular Affairs Frank McIntyre and severely criticized what they believed to be injustices committed against American nurses by Elsie McCloskey, chief nurse of Philippine General Hospital. Bruton accused McCloskey of insensitivity toward three American nurses who had become ill in the Philippines. Dugan complained of McCloskey's "tyrannical rule" that led to strained relations between the chief nurse and the twenty-five head nurses of the hospital.

In their letters, Bruton and Dugan highlighted incidents involving Filipino student nurses, claiming that McCloskey used Filipino student nurses in ways that insulted and degraded American nurses. For example, Bruton claimed that, after she had criticized McCloskey for the chief nurse's treatment of the ill American nurses, among the first ways McCloskey demonstrated her wrath was by ordering her "to move from the American nurses' home . . . and to take up [her] abode in the Filipino nurses' dormitory." Although Bruton was supposed to be the matron of that dormitory, McCloskey assigned her a small room, which, according to Bruton, "was directly over a pavilion that held all the garbage cans and refuse of the hospital."[47]

In Dugan's letter, she argued that the "climax" of the strained relations between McCloskey and the American head nurses occurred "when Miss McCloskey detailed a Filipina pupil nurse, to teach whom was one of the duties that brought us to the Islands, to supervise and inspect the American nurses' work." Given this order, Dugan continued, "naturally, all the American nurses felt highly incensed at this violation of ethics on the part of the chief nurse and the humiliation resulting therefrom, which made it impossible for the American nurses to maintain any kind of satisfactory discipline."[48]

These incidents reveal another complex angle of the interrelated nature of racialization and reform in American nursing in the colony. In the minds of Bruton and Dugan, teaching nursing to Filipinos may have been a moral obligation that exemplified America's humane imperialism. It was a duty that reflected a progressive element of the U.S. colonial nursing agenda to the extent that these nursing educators probably believed that it was indeed theoretically possible for Filipino nursing students to eventually become their professional equals. However, it was also a duty that assumed a temporal backwardness among Filipino student nurses. Filipino nursing students might become their equals sometime in the future but only through white American nurses' supervision and training.[49] Thus, for the time being, American nurses perceived living among Filipino nurses in their dormitory and working under their supervision as "naturally" humiliating.

AMERICAN DREAMS

Just as Lavinia Dock, Alice Bruton, and Mary Dugan interpreted nursing in the Philippines in vastly different ways, so too did the first Filipino student nurses. Excerpts of interviews with pioneering Filipino student nurses reveal that they interpreted the introduction of nursing in the archipelago as an opportunity to enter a new and prestigious profession that benefited Filipinos and the Philippine nation. The Philippine General Hospital School of Nursing would emphasize the link between nursing study and national service in their annual catalogue: "[Nursing] is a work that should appeal to every young Filipino man and woman of high aspirations, truly to serve their country."[50] Thus, Apolonia Salvador Ladao, one of the first graduates of the Philippine General Hospital School of Nursing, recalled, "When we took up nursing, we did not know what it was all about; we were simply selected and recommended by our American teachers. We were thankful of this opportunity to enter a new profession and to serve our people."[51]

These views of nursing dramatically contrast with historical interpretations that depict U.S. medical practices as racist and exploitive, illustrating the complexity of the meaning of nursing under U.S. colonialism. Professional nursing provided opportunities previously unavailable to young Filipino women. These included invitations to interact with colonial government officials and attend government functions. United States government officials may have showcased these nursing students as examples of Filipino potential and progress that had been "nurtured" under U.S. colonial rule, just as American organizers of world fairs' Philippine exhibits had done with the displays of U.S. colonial government-trained Philippine Scouts and Constabulary in the United States.[52] However, Filipino nursing students interpreted these opportunities as a form of prestige bestowed on them as a result of their study of nursing. Ramona Cabrera, another member of the first nursing class from Philippine General Hospital, explained, "I took up nursing without the slightest idea of the work. But when I was in, I found the work so interesting that now I can say that I would have been sorry if I were not a nurse. . . . The [American] people must have had a high regard for the work of nurses, as the high government officials were very kind and courteous to us. We were usually invited to accompany wives of the high government officials from Washington who were visiting the Islands. We were invited to the Governor-General's receptions and other important social functions."[53]

Nursing students were also afforded the opportunity to interact with students of medicine, a field from which they had been previously excluded, and from which prominent Filipinos such as Jose Rizal had emerged. As Veneranda Sulit-Atienza, one of the first nursing graduates of St. Luke's Hospital School of Nursing in 1911 recalled, "I had to work hard in order to keep up with class activities that seemed strange and difficult at first. I was particularly interested in the bacteriology class and was fascinated by the specimens our teacher showed us through the microscope. . . . The presence of normal school and premedic students in the same class made me feel proud and important."[54]

The closely linked opportunities of study abroad and professional advancement in the Philippines increased nursing's popularity. Beginning in 1913, the implementation of Governor-General Francis Burton Harrison's "Filipinization" campaign to replace American colonial government officials with Filipinos led to the appointment of Filipino nursing graduates to supervisory and faculty positions in Philippine hospitals and their schools of nursing. Anastacia Girón-Tupas, the first Filipino nurse to become the Philippine General Hospital's chief nurse and superintendent in the 1920s, was a 1917 graduate of the Pennsylvania School of Social Work. Her successor, Enriqueta Macaraig, graduated from Teachers College, Columbia University, in New York City in 1920.

The Filipinization of the nursing faculty at St. Luke's Hospital School of Nursing vividly illustrates the closely intertwined relationship between educational opportunities in the United States and professional advancement for nurses in the Philippines from the 1910s through the 1940s. In 1911, the first three graduates of St. Luke's Hospital School of Nursing, Quintana Beley, Veneranda Sulit, and Caridad Goco, completed their postgraduate coursework at Protestant Hospital in Philadelphia with financial assistance from the wife of a former U.S. ambassador to England. They returned to the Philippines and assumed faculty positions at St. Luke's. In 1922, the Rockefeller Foundation sponsored another St. Luke's graduate, Escolastica Agatep, to study at Columbia University's Teacher's College. Agatep returned to become the first Filipino nursing arts instructor at St. Luke's. In 1939, the Daughters of the American Revolution provided a scholarship to Imelda Tinawin, which supported her studies for the Bachelor of Science in Nursing Education from Columbia University. Upon her return to the Philippines, Tinawin held the position of principal of St. Luke's Hospital School of Nursing from 1943 to 1945. This process affected virtually all schools and later colleges of nursing in the Philippines. Study abroad in the United States became a de facto prerequisite for occupational mobility in the nursing profession in the Philippines.[55]

In addition to the individual sponsorship of Filipino nursing students by American individuals and foundations, the U.S. colonial government established a new education abroad program called the *pensionado* program.[56] Through this program the U.S. colonial government sponsored an elite group of male and female Filipino students called pensionados to study at U.S. colleges and universities. Colonial administrators expected the students to return to the Philippines and to assume positions in U.S.-established institutions. The U.S.-sponsored women students inspired some Filipino nurses to study abroad as well. In Patrocinio Montellano's case, a pensionada had reaffirmed her desire to go abroad. In the 1910s Montellano had wanted to see the United States by attending college abroad, but studied at the Philippine General Hospital School of Nursing; however, when her nursing classmate and close friend, Josefa Abaya, was able to study in the United States under the auspices of a U.S. colonial government scholarship, Montellano recollected that her "obsession to go abroad was rekindled." She insisted, "I was determined to follow her by all means."[57]

For the most part, however, American educational "opportunities" for Filipino women perpetuated America's gendered assumptions about labor, constructing the separate woman's sphere that many white American men and women of the period claimed to be one of the foundations for "civilization." Although Filipino women as well as men were able to study abroad as pensionados in the United States, the Filipino male students studied medicine and law, whereas the most popular fields of study for Filipino women in the United States were home economics, social and religious work, and nursing.[58] Some Filipino women students in the United States "invaded the sacred and hitherto exclusively men's realm of business and politics" through their studies abroad, but they were a minority.[59]

Furthermore, if Filipino nurses challenged the beliefs and authority of their American nursing supervisors, they too potentially earned the wrath of these women. For example, when Alice Fitzgerald of the Rockefeller Foundation International Health Board arrived in Manila in 1922 to survey the nursing situation in the colony, International Health Board Secretary Florence Reed advised Fitzgerald to develop a good relationship with Philippine General Hospital's chief nurse and supervisor Anastacia Girón. Fitzgerald initially characterized Girón as "very cooperative and friendly" and commented to Reed, "Of course, the fact that I like to work with and for natives does help." However, after Girón went against nursing school policy by marrying Dr. Albert Tupas, an instructor at the University of the Philippines College of Medicine and Surgery,

Fitzgerald supported Girón's resignation, claiming that "of course, a married woman cannot take the position of Superintendant of Nurses as that is certainly a full-time job." Fitzgerald interpreted Girón's "inexcusable behavior" as a threat to her professional accomplishments in the Philippines because, according to Fitzgerald, she had spent most of her time strengthening Girón's position. However, her feelings of uselessness and powerlessness among American male health officials in the Philippines offer another context for understanding her anger and disillusionment. During her tenure as a nursing consultant in the colony, Fitzgerald complained to the International Health Division General Director, "I do not feel that I am of any use whatever to the Governor General for he never refers anything to me either for my opinion or for advice."[60]

Finally, the specter of racism qualified the rosy depictions of nursing by some of the first Filipino nursing students. In her letter to Chief of Insular Affairs Frank McIntyre, Elsie McCloskey reported that racism had prevented Filipino nurses from doing some nursing work: "You can see by this what progress these little men and women have made in the Profession. We have twenty-four departments [in Philippine General Hospital] of which these young people are at the head of, except for three units — here we keep three American nurses for the exclusive care of American patients on account of the strong racial feeling, and not because the Filipino nurses can not do the work."[61] Even McCloskey's reference to Filipino nurses as "these little women and men" betrayed the racialized and gendered contrast between American patronage and Filipino childlike inferiority similarly assumed in the popular American reference to Filipinos as their "little brown brothers." In the gendered work of nursing, American women's tutelage of their "little brown sisters" illustrated that U.S. colonial agendas targeted Filipino women as well as men.

Yet, just as white American women used colonial nursing in their attempt to raise their status, so too did Filipino women. Some Filipino women used the work of Filipino nurses to promote a Philippine nationalist and feminist pride that importantly critiqued American ignorance of Filipino women's capabilities, but at the same time perpetuated stereotypical depictions of other Asian women as degraded sex objects at the disposal of Asian men. For example, in her 1920 article "Filipino Feminism," Emma Sarepta Yule situated Filipino feminism against a backdrop of Japanese and Indian women's oppression:

In an off-hand calculation the average American would place the Oriental Woman's value as a factor in the body politic very close to zero. Indeed, for him the phrase, "Oriental woman," conjures up only a weird sort of mental tapestry on which vague figures appear, some in mysterious veils through which gleam lustrous eyes, others with pitiful "lily-feet" showing below mannish trouser legs, flower like, others wearing absurd girdles, kneel on flat cushions, or stand with modest mien. . . . [This article] deals, however, with a woman of the East; but one who has not been presented to the Western world. . . . Lying midway between the dainty kimono of Japan and the veiled lady of India, and alongside of the "lily-footed" dame of China is the woman of the Philippines, a type of feminism unique in the Orient. A woman in whose development there has been neither seclusion, nor oppression, nor servitude.

Yule partly attributed this absence of oppression to her observation that "in the world's broad field of battle no sphere is closed to [the Filipino woman]." Her evidence for this observation was Filipino women's work in multiple fields, such as clerical work, teaching, and nursing. Yule wrote proudly that "the nurse's white cap is familiar in all larger towns."[62] The Filipino nurse's cap became the material expression of Filipino women's modernity, a symbol of their liberation that contrasted with the oppressive imagery of Japanese women's "dainty kimono," Indian women's "mysterious veils," and Chinese women's "mannish trouser legs." Ironically, such Filipino women's writing by Yule and others used strategies similar to those employed by white American women writers such as Lavinia Dock, who mistakenly characterized Filipino women as having the "same style of costume for about three hundred years."[63] Thus, if, as Joan Jacobs Brumberg pointed out, by 1900 white women had developed "an entire vocabulary that implied the degradation of [nonwhite, non-Western] women," a vocabulary that included harems, polygamy, and foot binding, so too had Filipino women writing in the 1920s, in ways that also used Asian women's oppression, but with the intention of uplifting their own status.[64]

Similar to Yule, other Filipino female self-proclaimed feminist writers, such as Encarnacion Alzona, the first Filipino woman to earn a doctorate of philosophy and author of the first published comprehensive history of Filipino women, argued that Filipino women were "unlike the women of other oriental countries." Alzona claimed that "they were never confined to a life of sheltered seclusion and ease." Furthermore, she continued, with the exception of the Mohammedans in Mindanao, the southern part of the archipelago, "the practice of monogamy distinguished the Filipinos from other oriental peoples." Although Alzona expressed gratitude to the U.S. colonial regime for the educational opportunities given to Filipino women, this gratitude did not mean that Americans had been responsible for Filipino women's high status.[65] Rather than attribute Filipino women's liberation to American tutelage, Alzona argued that the high status of Filipino women was part of an ancient Filipino heritage depicted by myths and legends, what another Filipino feminist writer, Paz Policarpio Mendez, would later refer to as "the high place occupied by Filipino women from *time immemorial.*"[66] This ancient Filipino heritage distinguished Filipinos, not only from other Asian countries, but also from the Western, Christian world. Alzona claimed:

> The ancient Filipinos were apparently aware of the equality of man and woman, for even in their legend about the origin of man this idea could be discerned. They believed that a large bird alighted on a huge bamboo and pecked at it so persistently that it was split open, and out of it emerged a man and woman who had never seen each other before, for they had lived in different joints of the bamboo. Upon beholding each other, the man bowed low before the woman, signifying the respect that man should pay to woman. Is not this legend very unlike the widely accepted Christian story of the creation of woman out of a rib of man, a story which is frequently cited to give an air of plausibility to the fallacious contention that woman is inferior to man by the very act of creation and therefore should be subject to man's authority. In a large measure the Biblical story of creation is responsible for the subjection of women for centuries throughout the Christian world as the laws of civilized countries alone reveal. Our Filipino legend at least traces the origin of man and woman to a common source, a bamboo, and thus places them on the same footing.[67]

Thus, in Alzona's depiction of Filipino women's history, the racialized evolutionary time line of progress assumed by white American women — in which primitive women could become civilized only under white American women's tutelage — did not apply to Filipino women. For Filipino women did not need to look to the present or future for civilization, but to their own civilized past.

Filipino nurses played a role in supporting Alzona's arguments. Alzona praised the medical efforts of the American colonial regime to end cholera and smallpox epidemics and to reduce the rate of infant mortality and the pervasiveness of tuberculosis. However, she pointed to the professional nursing work of Filipino women to emphasize that U.S. colonial officials could not have obtained achievements in public health without their cooperation and contributions: "The pioneer American public health officials in the Philippines realized the necessity of exterminating these enemies of progress and they guided the Filipinos in fighting them and improving public health in general. In their task, they were handicapped, however, by the lack of trained nurses. It was imperative, therefore, to enlist the cooperation of the Filipino women. At the beginning only a few women answered the call; but in later years, more and more of them were lured to the nursing profession. As the number of trained nurses increased, our government has been able to undertake important public health projects."[68]

The complex links among nursing, nationalism, and opportunities abroad for Filipino women had been established in the U.S. colonial period. These opportunities inspired some young Filipino women to take up the study of nursing and marked the beginning of their idealization of American work and academic experience. By 1916, Director of Education W. W. Marquardt reported that there were "over one thousand applications from intermediate girl graduates who desire to become nurses," with only fifty positions available at Philippine General Hospital.[69] In the 1910s, Filipino nursing student Patrocinio Montellano could dream to the point of obsession of seeing America. And by the early 1920s, some Filipino nurses studying abroad stayed in the United States for periods of time longer than U.S. colonial officials expected and desired. In 1921, William Musgrave (who had helped Montellano secure employment in the United States) wrote to Bureau of Insular Affairs educational agent Marquardt and reported with some alarm that Filipino nurses in San Francisco were choosing to remain there. He queried, "I am wondering whether you cannot in your official capacity assist in some way in getting these girls back to their own country and into the kind of work they have now been very well prepared to undertake."[70] Marquardt replied that, during his last visit to San Francisco, he had suggested to some of the Filipino nurses there to return to Manila, and concluded that "apparently my suggestions did not have much effect." He promised Musgrave that he would write to "a number of people in

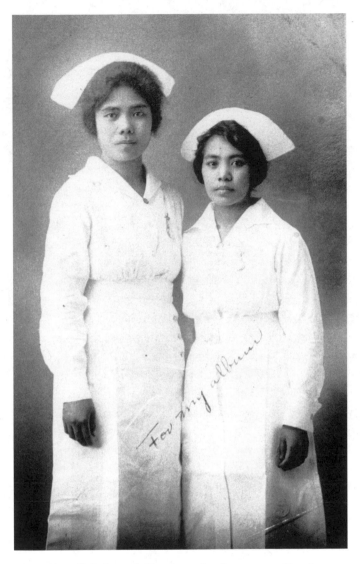

Maria Abastilla Beltran (left) prior to her departure to America in 1929. From Fred Cordova's *Filipinos: Forgotten Asian Americans*.

Manila in hopes of being able to bring enough influence to bear to secure the *desired* result."[71]

Some Filipino nurses who traveled to the United States to further their education did not come back to the Philippines, but settled permanently in the United States. In the 1920s, Maria Abastilla Beltran worked for the Philippine Chapter of the American Red Cross for four years. When asked if Americans in the Philippines had influenced her in any way, Beltran responded that she was close to Major Richards, a medical advisor to Governor-General Wood. She reminisced, "He saw my work in the Red Cross. He actually said to me, 'You know, Mary, if you went to the United States you could improve yourself very much. Mary, you are doing very good. . . . And you could be somebody else.'"[72] Partly as a result of his encouragement, Beltran planned to earn her B.A. in public health nursing in the United States and then return to the Philippines and resume working for the Red Cross there. However, after finishing her degree in 1931, she married a Filipino she had met in the United States and they settled in Seattle, Washington.

Although U.S. colonial officials attempted to implement their agendas in the Philippines, colonial changes produced unintended consequences, such as Filipino women's own strong desires to travel to the United States and to remain there indefinitely, and U.S. colonizers' inability to fully control Filipino women's mobility. Filipino nurses' idealization of American work and academic experience would be only one of several preconditions that would lay the foundation for Filipino nurse mass migrations overseas in the second half of the twentieth century. Americanized nursing education and work culture in the Philippines would inform and shape others.

CHAPTER 2

"The Usual Subjects"

The Preconditions of Professional Migration

As nonwhite and non-Western people opposed to Western medicine and nursing, and as native bodies full of dangerous germs, Filipinos, like Africans and Indians, were the usual subjects of colonial control by Western nations, in this case, the United States. However, "the usual subjects" also signified the Americanized theoretical and practical training of Filipino nurses during the U.S. colonial period. Lavinia Dock described the original curriculum of the first government-sponsored Filipino nursing students: "A thorough course of study was arranged, including, besides all *the usual subjects,* the nursing of tropical diseases, the sanitary work of the Bureau of Health, public instruction in dispensary and school work, English grammar and colloquial English, and industrial and living conditions in the islands."[1]

Although some scholars have acknowledged the historical relationship between late twentieth-century Filipino nurse migrations to the United States and early twentieth-century American colonial educational policies (including Americanized nursing education) in the Philippines, their analyses of this relationship leave many questions unanswered: What exactly did an Americanized nursing education entail? How did it prepare Filipino nurses to work abroad in the United States?[2] I argue that the contemporary international migration of Filipino nurses is inextricably linked to early twentieth-century U.S. colonialism in the Philippines because important preconditions that enabled this form of professional migration were established under the U.S. colonial regime. In addition to the idealization of U.S. work and academic experience that I discussed in the previous chapter, these preconditions included (1) Americanized professional nursing training, (2) English-language fluency, (3) Americanized nursing work culture, and (4) gendered notions of nursing as women's work. These preconditions created a Filipino labor force with the labor skills, professional credentials, and

English-language ability necessary to work in U.S. hospitals as well as a labor force accustomed to the work culture of these institutions. They would lay the foundation for a gendered, racialized, and professional labor force prepared for export to the United States in the tens of thousands by the 1950s through the present.

This chapter examines the development of these preconditions, beginning with the U.S. colonial government's institutionalization of nursing training in 1907, through the professionalization of Philippine nursing in the 1920s and 1930s, and concluding with the persistence of U.S. colonial nursing patterns even after Philippine independence in 1946. Although this chapter's detailed analysis of this development traces the ways Philippine nursing was informed by and chronologically followed U.S. professional nursing trends, American nursing was "never self-evidently hegemonic," nor was it seamlessly reproduced in the archipelago.[3] Rather, the professional development of Philippine nursing under U.S. colonial rule was an ongoing process that had been shaped by both Filipino and American nurses. Furthermore, in the first half of the twentieth century, the profession of nursing was undergoing major transformation on both sides of the ocean, in the United States as well as the Philippines. The dynamics of Philippine *and* American nursing precluded monolithic definitions of nursing work in both countries, and thus prevented simplistic reproductions of American nursing in the Philippines.

AMERICANIZED SUBJECTS

The construction of an Americanized nursing curriculum in the Philippines was one of the most significant preconditions for the mass migration of Filipino nurses in the late twentieth century. From 1907 to 1910, the training of the first Filipino nursing students began with a common first year of classroom study at the Philippine Normal School. The student nurses then separated for their practical nursing work at three different hospital schools of nursing: St. Paul's Hospital, the Civil Hospital (later known as Philippine General Hospital), and University Hospital (later known as St. Luke's Hospital). This arrangement was a practical one because these hospitals and their corresponding schools of nursing were just getting underway; by 1910, however, Filipino nursing students completed both their classroom and practical nursing work in their individual hospitals, as was the practice in the United States.

The first Filipino nursing students studied the usual subjects of practical nursing, materia medica, massage, and bacteriology. They also heard lectures on medicine, communicable diseases, and operating room techniques. By 1915, the curriculum of Philippine General Hospital School of Nursing had been organized into thirteen departments: general nursing; anatomy; physiology; pharmacy and materia medica; bacteriology and clinical laboratory; obstetrics; pediatrics; surgery; medicine; eye, ear, nose, and throat; hygiene; graduate courses; and a special midwifery course.[4] General nursing included subjects such as massage, hospital housekeeping, ethics, and hospital records.

From the beginning of U.S. colonial government-sponsored nursing training, as Dock's description of the curriculum mentions, the study of English (grammar as well as colloquial English) was an integral part of nursing students' curriculum. This English-language component of their training was one of the more unique aspects of American colonial education in general and medical training in particular. By contrast, David Arnold notes in his history of state medicine and epidemic disease in nineteenth-century India that the training of Indian doctors in British colonial India's Native Medical Institution was initially conducted in the vernacular and Western medical texts were translated for Indian students.[5] According to Rita Headrick's study on colonialism, health, and illness in French Equatorial Africa from 1885 to 1935, no systematic attempt was made to teach African nurses, many of whom were illiterate, to read or write.[6] In the Philippines, however, a representative from the Bureau of Education offered English instruction once a week over two and a half years to students of the Philippine General Hospital School of Nursing.[7] Although Spanish was also a mandatory part of the nursing curriculum over two and a half years, it would not become part of the nursing board examination. By contrast, in the 1920 Philippine board examination for nurses, English comprised 5 percent of the first part of the examination, along with nursing subjects such as anatomy, physiology, urinalysis, and dietetics.[8]

Aside from the usual subjects and the study of English, the early training of Filipino nurses followed other patterns of early twentieth-century U.S. nursing training in the United States, patterns that reflected the gendered, classed, and sexualized social order of American professional

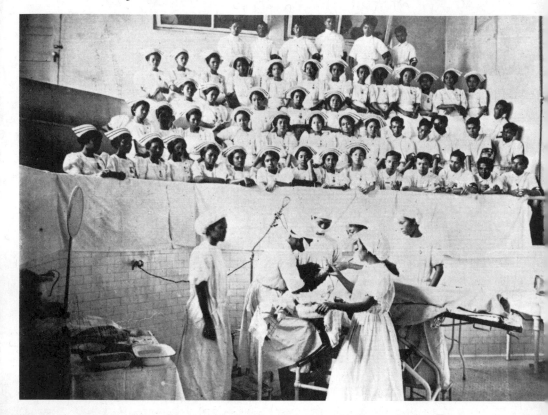

"Senior class receiving instruction in operating-room techniques, Philippine General Hospital" from Philippine General Hospital School of Nursing Ninth Annual Announcement and Catalogue, 1915–1916. U.S. National Archives, College Park, Maryland.

nursing. First, the U.S. colonial government attempted to legislate the creation of a female nursing labor force through a 1909 act that appropriated funds for classes comprising "Filipino women students."[9] As Dock noted in her history of Philippine nursing, the original nursing force under U.S. colonial rule disrupted American hospital habits through its use of Filipino male attendants to care for male patients. The first graduating classes of Philippine General Hospital School of Nursing in 1911 and 1912 consisted of six and thirty-five female students, respectively.

Second, the first U.S. nursing schools in the Philippines recruited young women from "respectable" families. In the United States in the mid–nineteenth century, nursing was primarily the work of white, native-born, poor, and older women who entered nursing at the end of their working lives, often for lack of other options. Hospital nurses during this period were often former patients of their hospital, as the prevalence of cross-infection within hospitals made recruitment of nurses difficult. Inspired by the work of Florence Nightingale, American nursing leaders tried to reform the image of nursing through the hospital training schools for nurses first established in 1873.[10] They aimed to reform nursing into suitable employment for young "gentlewomen" with the virtues and qualities of middle- and upper-class womanhood in Victorian America. In the Philippines in the early 1900s, the first nursing schools followed these American nursing reforms by also recruiting young women from respectable Filipino families. St. Paul's Hospital, Philippine General Hospital, and St. Luke's Hospital selected nursing students with the following qualifications: "good and sound physical mental health, good moral character, good family and social standing, and recommendations from three different persons well known in the community."[11]

Third, imperative to the recruitment of young Filipino gentlewomen from respectable families was the creation of the "protected environment" of the hospital. In the United States, American nursing leaders aimed to transform the hospital training school into a protected environment for young female nursing students managed by a "hospital family."[12] U.S. hospital schools of nursing recruited young women from rural areas to their hospitals, which functioned as safe havens in urban areas.[13] Similarly, the first Philippine schools of nursing recruited young Filipino women from areas as far as Cebu in the Visayas (the middle region of the archipelago) to train in their hospitals in Manila in Luzon (the northern region).[14] Although some of the first Filipino nursing students traveled far from their families, they also lived in the protected environment of a special dormitory. The dormitory opened in 1906 for Filipino female students enrolled in the Philippine Normal School, upon the urging of Mary Coleman. Young Filipino women living there, including the first nursing students, learned "social graces" and methods of "home management."[15] American and Filipino advocates for the first training schools for Filipino nurses acted as members of a hospital family. As Sofia de Veyra related, "We did a lot of *mothering* to the first girls and used a great deal of diplomacy and tact to keep them going and keeping up their interest in their work."[16]

Finally, from the early twentieth century to the 1950s, Filipino nursing students shared a similar work culture with American nursing students in the United States. In both countries, schools of nursing required that student nurses live in the hospital's nursing residence.[17] American and Filipino nursing students worked and resided within hospital grounds under the close supervision of hospital superintendents and matrons. The strict discipline and hard physical work of nursing training, inspired by Nightingale's vision of models of hierarchy, duty, and discipline from the military and the Victorian family, bonded American nursing students in the United States. It also brought Filipino nursing students together. Purita Asperilla described her nursing training at the Philippine General Hospital in the late 1930s: "You tend to become close to your friends, your classmates, because you live together. You sleep together. Our matron was very strict. . . . Nursing as [a] profession before the war, World War II, was militaristic. You have to arrange your clothes this way. . . . And they inspect you every morning before you go to the hall. They inspect you [to see] whether you have holes in your stockings. And your hair should be cropped like this. You cannot hang your hair."[18]

Furthermore, throughout the first half of the twentieth century, American and Philippine hospital schools of nursing depended on the labor of their nursing students. The study of nursing was in many ways an extension of rigorous and intensive domestic work in a hospital setting. Nursing student duties included washing operating sheets and towels and scrubbing bathroom floors. By 1900, terms like "hospital machine" and "industrial slave" were used to describe the American student nurse. In the United States, hospital training schools used nursing students as an inexpensive source of labor, providing them with board and lodging and small allowances, which in the early 1900s and 1910s averaged $8 to $12 a month.[19]

In the Philippines, the duties of Filipino nursing students were very similar and their compensation also minimal. Purita Asperilla related, "You see, at that time, our education was done in the morning, then we are on duty in the afternoon. We are depended upon for service. . . . There were times when we were assigned in the morning. But you know, the first part of the curriculum is no hospital work. We were in the linen room. We were arranging linens, mending linens, torn linens. We fold linens. I think that was one month. And then after that we were assigned to the clinical areas."[20]

These forms of labor were incorporated and legitimized in the Philippine nursing curriculum as the study of "hospital housekeeping," which entailed instruction "in the care and issuing of supplies; methods of cleaning buildings, equipment, and furniture; care and handling of linen and laundry; economy in the use of supplies; and other phases of house-keeping." According to the 1915 catalogue of the Philippine General Hospital School of Nursing, nursing students received board and lodging and a monthly allowance of 16 pesos during the preliminary year of study, 18 pesos during the junior year, and 20 pesos during the senior year. As in the United States, the allowance was supposed to cover the costs of students' laundry, uniform, books, and other equipment. The Philippine General Hospital School of Nursing catalogue indirectly denied the exploitation of students' labor by emphasizing that the allowance was in no way a form of salary, "the professional education being considered sufficient additional compensation."[21]

Although Filipino nursing students studied some of the same subjects as American nursing students, the early twentieth-century nursing curriculum in the Philippines was never a mirror-image reproduction of the American nursing curriculum in the United States. As Dock's history noted, the first Filipino nursing students studied "the nursing of tropical diseases" and "industrial and living conditions in the islands," subjects more relevant to nursing students in the Philippines. American colonial intentions of remaking Filipinos in their own image through assimilationist techniques, such as the study of English and the adoption of American medical practices, also developed in uneven ways. Filipino nurses' study of English did not translate into a loss of their first language. Rather, Philippine schools of nursing believed that Filipino health could "best be accomplished through the specialized [nursing] education of a selected number who will then spread their knowledge in *the dialects of their own people.*"[22]

Furthermore, the enrollment of Filipino male students in hospital schools of nursing disrupted the American female-gendered work culture of nursing. Although Dock had written about an attempt to remove men from the nursing labor force by segregating them in a separate training school, and although the 1909 Act appropriating funds for nursing classes specifically referred to the recruitment of Filipino female students, Philippine General Hospital School of Nursing catalogues from 1915–1916 and 1917–1918 depicted Filipino male nursing students and supervisors as an integral part of the school. Although the six nursing graduates from the first class of 1911 and the thirty-five graduates from the class of 1912 were all female, the graduates of the class of 1913 included twenty-seven women and twenty-six men. In the class of 1914, thirty-six graduates were women and sixteen were men.[23] In addition, by 1916, Filipino men comprised a significant percentage of nursing supervisors (six out of twenty-seven) and head nurses (nine out of thirty-nine) at Philippine General Hospital.[24] The hospital's nursing school catalogues also revealed the active inclusion of men in the school's recruitment of nurses and its awarding of honors and prizes. In its requirements for admission, "unmarried Filipinos, *both male and female*, over 18 1/2 years of age" with satisfactory educational, physical, and moral qualifications were eligible to apply. At graduation the school of nursing presented a gold medal to "the student of each sex" with the highest general record.[25]

The catalogues did not explain why this gendered shift took place in the midst of U.S. colonial rule and despite colonial efforts to impose a different, strictly female-gendered labor force. Its depictions suggest only that the imposition of American gendered norms in the Philippine colony was contested and incomplete. Even in the United States, the "women's" work of nursing included a minority of men. As early as 1900, an article in *Nursing Record* by a male nurse trained at Bellevue Hospital in New York described the "training of male nurses."[26] In her study of the early twentieth-century Rockefeller Foundation agenda in Philippine nursing, Barbara Brush suggests that some American nurses in the Philippines, such as Alice Fitzgerald, reluctantly agreed to include Filipino male nurses, especially in fields such as public health nursing in which, according to Fitzgerald, "there are many isolated districts where it would not be right to send a young woman and where the male nurses can do good work."[27]

Nevertheless, the awarding of two medals (one for "each sex") and the listing of nursing graduates by "male" and "female" graduates, reflected both the inclusion of men in the nursing school as well as an awareness and acknowledgment of sex difference. Although female and male nursing students completed the same coursework and trained in the same classrooms together, the Philippine General Hospital School of Nursing designated separate assistant principals (one male and one female) for the "male school of nursing" and "female school of nursing."[28] Photographs of student nurses' athletic classes and teams also presented separate female and male groups.

Furthermore, although the strict surveillance of both male and female students' behavior was an integral part of the work culture of nursing, more rules and regulations governed women's (both student nurses and graduate nurses) actions. By contrast, male students were given some privileges. Under its section on "Rules for Dormitories," the 1923 Philippine General Hospital *Manual for Nurses* outlined the guidelines for proper behavior: "No graduate nurse not on duty shall be out of the dormitory after 9 p.m. and no student after 6 p.m. *except the male students* who shall not be allowed to go out after 7 p.m. during school days. *Female nurses and students shall not go out alone at any time.* They may go in couples or in large parties of the same sex. When in company of male friends there shall be, at all times, an extra female companion present who shall act as chaperon. Student nurses can not act as chaperon. A number of graduate nurses shall be selected from time to time by the chief nurse to act as chaperons to female pupil nurses when going out."[29]

Finally, although the 1915–16 and 1916–17 annual catalogues of the Philippine General Hospital School of Nursing showed that Filipino male students comprised a significant percentage of the school's graduating classes after 1912, female students consistently outnumbered them, suggesting that the process of feminizing the nursing labor force was underway. Furthermore, increasing antimale sentiments by the American-run Red Cross and Public Welfare Commission threatened the employment of male graduates in the field of public health nursing.[30] Over the next two decades, Filipino women emerged at the helm of Philippine nursing leadership.

THE PROCESS OF PROFESSIONALIZATION

In the 1920s and 1930s, Philippine schools of nursing continued to adopt trends of American professional nursing, such as higher standards of admission, the specialization of public health nursing, and the formation of nursing organizations. In the United States, growing concerns over nursing educational standards paralleled the history of the professionalization of American nursing. Nursing alumni associations formed in the 1880s and 1890s transformed into professional nursing organizations, the National League of Nursing Education and the American Nurses Association. Among other issues, American professional nursing leaders

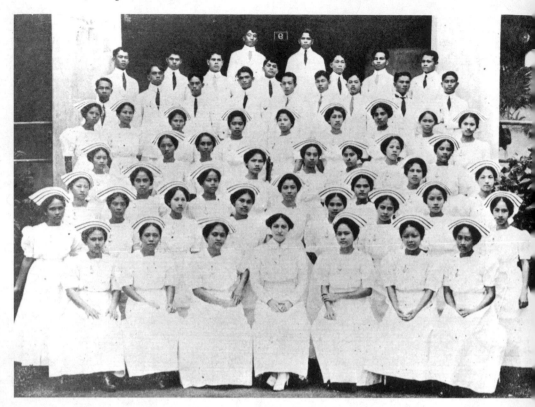

"1915 class and the Superintendent of the School of Nursing, Philippine General Hospital" from Philippine General Hospital School of Nursing Ninth Annual Announcement and Catalogue, 1915–1916. U.S. National Archives, College Park, Maryland.

preoccupied themselves with raising nursing educational standards in the belief that such requirements and restrictions would not only regulate the oversupply of nurses but also increase nursing autonomy and prestige. Raising nursing educational standards involved measures such as the reduction of the number of nursing schools and more stringent entrance requirements.

Historians Barbara Melosh and Susan Reverby have pointed out that many working nurses in the United States, who were being excluded by the educational reform of professional nursing leaders, contested these professionalizing efforts.[31] In the late nineteenth and early twentieth centuries, American nursing underwent major conflict as well as change. However, educational changes in Philippine nursing schools followed the pattern of American *professional* nursing. In 1907, entrance require-ments of the first government training school for Filipino nurses in-cluded a minimum educational preparation of completion of the seventh grade and a qualifying examination.[32] The largest hospital school of nursing, Philippine General Hospital, raised its entrance requirements in 1917, requiring the completion of the first year of secondary school for admission. Only one year later, completion of the second year became a prerequisite. In 1926, entrance requirements included completion of the third year. Four years later, the completion of secondary school was required for admission. By 1933, Philippine General Hospital School of Nursing gave preference for admission to those Filipino applicants who had completed six units of credit in the University of the Philippines College of Liberal Arts. Other Philippine schools of nursing raised their educational entrance requirements accordingly.[33]

In the United States, the specialization of public health nursing emerged during a 1912 American Nurses Association convention when sixty-nine nurses established a National Organization for Public Health Nursing.[34] The field experienced its height of popularity from the 1920s to 1950s. Focusing on preventive work and "positive health," public health nurses worked outside the more traditional nursing contexts of private duty and hospital work through visiting nurses' associations, settlement houses, child welfare associations, and factory dispensaries, thereby expanding medical intervention in various areas of work, leisure, and general daily living.

In the Philippines, the rise of public health nursing followed a similar chronology. The first Filipino public health nurses worked in child wel-fare centers, health centers, and dispensaries throughout the Philippines. In 1912, the Bureau of Health employed four graduates of the Philippine General Hospital School of Nursing in maternal and child health work in Cebu City and nearby towns.[35] In 1914, these nurses cared for nearly three thousand patients primarily through house visits. In the province of Albay, three public health nurses served 10,400 public school children at 124 public schools. In the city of Malolos, Bulacan, three public health nurses provided nursing care to children and to prospective mothers. According to one report, "Natives who are afraid of hospitals and doc-tors call for the [public health] nurses."[36]

Along with school textbooks, the local press, Bureau of Health bul-letins, and the Bureau's lecture and exhibit car, Filipino public health nurses helped to transform Filipinos' daily practices and attitudes about health outside of a hospital setting. The visibility of public health nurses also presented new career possibilities for Filipino children. Before Purita Asperilla studied nursing at Philippine General Hospital in the 1930s, she claimed that her brothers and sisters teased her about wanting to become a nurse. Yet she was undeterred by their taunts: "I said, I don't mind. I was very much impressed by my school nurse and I was recruited to be in the nutrition program. As a child, I was very sports-minded. In fact, I belonged to a team. . . . So I was in the nutrition clinic and we were given milk. The nurse was very close to us. She took our weight, put us to sleep during recess time. This nurse would give us a gold star if we gained two pounds, a silver star if you gained one pound."[37]

As in the United States, public health nursing in the Philippines became increasingly specialized. In 1922, the Philippine Health Service in cooperation with the University of the Philippines, the Philippine General Hospital, the Public Welfare Commission, the Philippine Chapter of the American Red Cross, and other philanthropic organizations established the first course to train Filipino nurses in public health nursing. By 1938, the Philippines had its first college graduates of the School of Public Health Nursing at the University of the Philippines.[38]

The efforts of the first Filipino nurse graduates enabled the development of these professional nursing trends. They organized themselves at a meeting that led to the establishment of a Philippine professional nursing organization with Filipino nursing leadership. Although Barbara Brush's study claims that this meeting was the result of Alice Fitzgerald's suggestion (based on letters and reports written by Fitzgerald), Filipino accounts acknowledge Fitzgerald's guidance without attributing the idea of the formation of a Philippine professional nursing organization to her alone. In 1922, Anastacia Girón-Tupas and 150 Filipino graduate nurses convened to organize the Filipino Nurses Association (FNA). They elected Rosario Montenegro Delgado, graduate of the Philippine General Hospital nursing class of 1912, to be its first president. Alice Fitzgerald served as advisor to the FNA. In addition, American nurses, including Fitzgerald and Lillian Weiser (chief nurse and superintendent of St. Luke's Hospital), participated as honorary members.[39]

Through the FNA, Filipino nurses increased educational standards of nursing training, developed the practice and training of public health nurses, and engaged in other nursing activities similar to those of professional nursing organizations in Europe and the United States. Its overall purpose was "to exalt the standard of the nursing profession and other allied purposes."[40] The FNA created the League of Nursing Education, which published standard nursing curriculums, raised admission requirements to Philippine schools of nursing, and advocated a baccalaureate program in nursing. In 1924, the League published its first standard curriculum for schools of nursing. In 1932, it raised and standardized Philippine nursing schools' minimum educational requirements for admission to the completion of secondary school. The FNA's first resolution was a petition for the creation of a College of Nursing at the University of the Philippines.

Another allied purpose of the FNA, "to cooperate with other organizations in the reduction of infant mortality and in the repression of preventable diseases in the Philippines Islands," promoted public health nursing in the Philippines. Public health nursing, along with nursing education and private nursing, comprised the first three sections of the FNA. During the FNA's first annual meeting in January, a major objective of the public health nursing section was the establishment of a Philippine nursing journal, which would devote a section to public health nursing news.[41] The FNA published the first issue of the *Message of the Public Health Nurse* in October 1924. In 1926, the *Filipino Nurse* replaced the *Message* as the official publication of the FNA. In 1953, the FNA renamed the publication as the *Philippine Journal of Nursing*.

U.S. professional nursing continued to be a dominant force in Philippine nursing's development through the 1930s. However, this development was not a simple transfer of nursing ideas from the United States to the Philippines by Americans to Filipinos. Travel arrangements enabled Filipino nurses to study nursing trends in the United States and then institute those changes they deemed relevant and appropriate. Filipino nurse graduates who were able to pursue postgraduate study in the United States returned to the Philippines to perpetuate American nursing trends. For example, in 1939, the secretary of public instruction appointed a committee to revise the Philippine nursing curriculum. A subcommittee of Filipino nurses who had recently returned from the United States in 1945 reviewed the proposed new curriculum so that it would be "consistent with the latest trends in higher education abroad."[42]

Aside from its focus on nursing education and public health, and the publication of its own nursing journal, the FNA shared other organizational similarities with professional nursing organizations around the world. It registered Filipino nurses, created a central directory for private duty employment, advocated increased salaries for nurses and a government nurses' pension, provided financial assistance to elderly and sick nurses, and started scholarship funds for nursing students. These activities helped the FNA gain membership in the International Council of Nurses (ICN) in 1929. British nursing leaders organized the ICN in 1899; its first members were national nurses associations from Great Britain, Ireland, the United States, and Germany. One national nursing association composed of trained nurses for each country was eligible for ICN membership provided that its constitution and by-laws promoted the objectives of the ICN. Among the ICN's aims were raising the standards of nursing education and promoting professional ethics and the public usefulness of its members.

The global vision espoused by the ICN helped to transform nursing into an international profession. In the preamble of the ICN Constitution, adopted in 1900, members proclaimed that, as "nurses of all nations," they believed that "the best good of our Profession will be advanced by greater unity of thought, sympathy, and purpose." Their major objectives, as stated in the first article of the constitution, were "to provide a means of communication between the Nurses of all Nations, and to afford facilities for the interchange of international hospitality" and "to provide opportunities for nurses to meet together from all parts of the world." The ICN continued to internationalize the nursing profession in the 1910s and 1920s by defining standards for professional nursing education ("a minimum of three years' continuous training in recognised qualified training schools . . . under the direction of a trained nurse or professional superintendent") and determining a definition for the trained nurse ("a nurse who during her training has received instruction and experience in at least four of the main branches of nursing, including medical, surgical, and children's nursing, and who is prepared on graduation to enter the general practice of nursing").[43] By the time of the FNA's admission into the ICN in 1929, Philippine nursing education and Filipino trained nurses had met these standards.

Colonialism was only one of many geopolitical forces that complicated the seemingly neutral dynamics of an international community of nurses, a community in which its national members supposedly convened as equals. Nurses from North American and European countries, primarily from Great Britain and the United States, dominated the leadership and proceedings of the ICN. Although the ICN theoretically supported "opportunities for nurses to meet together from all parts of the world," even its meeting places for its international congresses predominantly took place in European and North American countries, compelling delegates of the FNA to travel greater distances. Thus, the FNA offered to host the 1937 ICN congress in the Philippines with a rhetoric that carefully paid respect to European and North American ICN leaders: "The most humble greetings from members of our Association. Our imagination of the Congress is indeed great; and we look forward to the real living growth and vigorous advance of the knowledge and ideals which you eminent representatives of different nations are unselfishly working for and unceasingly contributing to the welfare of nurses all the world over. Paris, Brussels, London, Copenhagen and Montreal are in *far-away countries!* May it be possible for consideration that the next International Congress of Nurses take place at the "Pearl of the Orient Seas"—Manila, the Philippine Islands?"[44] However, the National Council of Nurses of Great Britain had also offered to host the 1937 congress and received the highest number of votes. Ethel Gordon Bedford Fenwick of Great Britain, the major founder of the ICN, had emphasized that twenty-five years had passed since the congress had last been held in London.

World War II and the Japanese occupation of the Philippines in 1942 violently disrupted training and practice at the hospital schools of nursing in Manila. Although training continued at some institutions, such as Philippine General Hospital and St. Luke's Hospital, according to Josefina Sablan, who studied at St. Luke's from 1939 until 1942, the Japanese regime compelled them to train under a Japanese principal and to study the Japanese language.[45] In her history of Philippine nursing, Anastacia Girón-Tupas detailed the destructive impact of the war at individual Philippine hospitals. During the American seige of South Manila in 1945, more than ten thousand refugees occupied the wards, basement, dispensary, and all other available spaces at Philippine General Hospital. Girón-Tupas recounted, "Some of them were hit by shrapnel and were instantly killed. The hospital became a virtual battleground as bullets from both the Americans and Japanese were exchanged. But the doctors and nurses stood their grounds and performed their sacred duties in the face of dangers."[46] Among the wounded graduate nurses were Avelina

Zalameda, Bienvenido Salvo, Concepcion Ballesteros, Juliana Torralba, Prima Llamas, Epigenia Racela, Lorenza Manzanilla, and Filomena Guerrero. Among the wounded student nurses were Gloria Castello, Eufronia Duruin, and Socorro Trinidad. The American Philippine War Damage Commission was able to rebuild Philippine General Hospital after the war. However, St. Paul's Hospital, located in Intramuros, the scene of a fierce battle between Japanese and American forces, like many other buildings in that area did not survive the war.

In 1947, thirty-two Filipino delegates and observers attended the first post–World War II congress of the ICN held in New York City. During a session presided by Filipino delegate Julita Sotejo, a delegate from Great Britain moved that delegates from all over the world stand for one minute in silent tribute to the achievements and struggles of Filipino nurses during the war. This moment reflected the international nursing community's recognition of the work of Filipino nurses as well as the recent independence of the Philippines from the United States in 1946.

Nevertheless, some U.S. colonial patterns in Philippine nursing education persisted after independence. Filipino nurses continued to follow trends of professional nursing in the United States, such as the popularization of the baccalaureate degree in nursing. In the United States, university schools of nursing emerged in the 1920s offering baccalaureate degrees in nursing, although four-year nursing programs did not become a trend until the late 1940s. In the Philippines between 1946 and 1948, nine universities and colleges began to offer baccalaureate programs in nursing.[47]

In the late 1940s, American philanthropic organizations continued to sponsor Filipino nursing graduates to study abroad. In 1948, Purita Asperilla earned her master's degree in nursing from Case Western University funded by a fellowship from China Medical Board, a subsidiary of the Rockefeller Foundation.[48] She returned to the Philippines and organized the college of nursing at the University of the East's Ramon Magsaysay Memorial Medical Center. According to Asperilla the medical center's administrators wanted her to organize a diploma program, but she successfully advocated a baccalaureate program that included two years of liberal arts studies and three years of clinical training.[49]

In the late 1940s, the Filipino nurses who traveled to the United States continued to be few in number. For the majority of Filipino nurses who were graduating from diploma as well as baccalaureate programs in larger numbers, going abroad to the United States was only a dream. However, in 1948, the U.S. government established the Exchange Visitor Program. This program would transform that dream of going abroad into a dream come true.

PART II

Caring Unbound

Dear Nurse: . . . We have placed over 8,000 nurses to different parts of the world. . . . So if you're not happy wherever you are right now, why not take the easy way out and go someplace else. We can't promise you'll find happiness, but we can help you chase it all over the place.
— Nurse recruitment advertisement for Manila Educational & Exchange Placement Service, *Philippine Journal of Nursing* 34.5 (September–October 1965)

I got carried on the wave of the gang, like a cohort of friends wanting to come to the United States for adventure, fun. . . . We go to parties and all you hear is, "Oh, there's this recruiting agency!"
— Filipino nurse ROSARIO-MAY MAYOR, reminiscing about her decision to immigrate to the United States in the early 1970s, interview with author, November 18, 1994, New York City

It is a paradox; we have no shortage of nurses but we lack nurses. . . . are we educating the nurses for home consumption or exportation?
— ROSARIO S. DIAMANTE, dean of Philippine Women's University College of Nursing, "Nursing Education in the Philippines Today," 1972

CHAPTER 3

"Your Cap Is a Passport"

Filipino Nurses and the U.S. Exchange Visitor Program

The establishment of an Americanized training hospital system in the Philippines during the U.S. colonial period created the professional, social, and cultural foundations that enabled a Filipino nursing labor force to work in the United States. Furthermore, given the complex histories of Spanish and U.S. colonization of the Philippines, Filipino women in general and Filipino nurses specifically viewed work and study in the United States as a desirable experience, a prestigious path to professional mobility on their return to the Philippines. These factors are important historical linkages that connect early twentieth-century colonization with the mass migration of Filipino nurses to the United States in the post-1965 period. Yet, new questions emerge: How did overseas work and study in the United States transform from an opportunity for the Philippine nursing elite in the early twentieth century into a *mass* migration of Filipino nurses in the post-1965 period? Furthermore, if study and work in the United States had become a path for professional mobility on Filipino nurses' return to the Philippines in the early twentieth century, why did so many Filipino nurses *immigrate* to the United States through the occupational preference categories of the Immigration Act of 1965? Why did significant numbers of Filipino nurses in the late twentieth century desire to remain in the United States as a more permanent part of the American nursing labor force, and not return to the Philippines?

The numerical, socioeconomic, and cultural significance of migration abroad for Filipino nurses changed dramatically in the mid–twentieth century. Epifanio Mercado's story illustrates some of these complex changes. Epi (as she preferred to be called) immigrated to the United States in 1971. When asked if her work as a nurse in the United States was what she had expected, she responded that she was already accustomed to working in the United States.[1] Mercado first came to the

United States in 1961 under the auspices of the U.S. Exchange Visitor Program (EVP). A friend who was also involved in the program encouraged her to come to the United States and even helped her with the paperwork. According to Mercado, although she wanted to visit the United States, she was not overly enthusiastic about the idea. However, exchange visitors were supposed to stay in the United States for a maximum of two years, after which they would return to their country of origin.

After working and studying in New York City as an exchange visitor nurse, Mercado claimed that she liked living in the United States. Her salary as an exchange nurse was higher than her earnings as a nurse in the Philippines, enabling her to help her family financially. "In the Philippines," she explained, "your salary is just enough for you." She also preferred the United States over the Philippines "culturally": "You can go to Broadway, Lincoln Center. You have enough money to travel. There's always something going on."

Instead of returning to the Philippines after the expiration of her exchange visa, Mercado exited the United States by going to Canada and then returned to New York in an attempt to resettle there. However, given the rules and regulations of the EVP at the time, she was unable to apply for an immigrant visa in New York City. She returned to the Philippines in 1969 to apply for an immigrant visa, and then went back to the United States after a wait of two years.

In the mid–twentieth century, exchange programs acted as vehicles for transforming nursing into an international profession. This chapter explores Filipino nurse migration to the United States in the 1950s and 1960s through the EVP and analyzes the complex social, economic, and cultural changes surrounding this form of migration. These changes included, first, the creation of new desires among the Filipino exchange nurses. Although some of them, like Mercado, were initially ambivalent about working in the United States, Filipino exchange nurses came to appreciate working abroad because that experience—the travel, professional opportunity, earnings, material accumulation, and leisure that accompanied it—translated into a unique form of socioeconomic success in the Philippines. Second, the prestige associated with the new lifestyle of Filipino exchange nurses changed the culture of Filipino nurse migration abroad. Instead of earning U.S. educational credentials and returning to work in the Philippines, subsequent generations of Filipino nursing graduates aimed to live abroad indefinitely. For young Filipino women, nursing opportunities abroad, and not in their home country, became motivations for engaging in the study of nursing in the first place. As a result, Filipino nurses, along with Filipino recruiters and U.S. hospital administrators, transformed the EVP into an avenue for the first wave of Filipino nurse mass migration into the United States.

Controversial debates regarding nursing and nationalism accompanied these changes. These controversies only hint at the numerous complexities, mythologies, and contradictions embedded in the EVP. In the Philippines, the prestige associated with work abroad fueled Filipino nurses' desire to migrate overseas despite troubling reports of U.S. hospital exploitation. Philippine government and health officials expressed intense pride as well as prejudice against the Filipino exchange nurse. In the United States, the absence of professional solidarity between American and Filipino nurses led some Filipino exchange nurses to align with exploitive hospital employers in their desire to remain abroad. In both countries, the program promoted nationalist agendas in the context of international exchange.

This chapter highlights these complexities and contradictions by historically connecting this unique form of migration to both early twentieth-century nurse migrations during the U.S. colonial period and later twentieth-century migrations of Filipino nurses to the United States. I argue, first, that Filipino exchange nurse migration refashioned, yet also perpetuated, the social and racialized hierarchies created by U.S. colonialism in the Philippines. Second, the transnational dynamics of Filipino exchange nurse migration, which took place in the context of U.S. attempts to maintain its global dominance during the cold war, prefigured the post-1965 immigration of Filipino nurses to the United States that so many studies have attributed solely to the "liberalization" of U.S. immigration laws, and specifically the passage of the U.S. Immigration Act of 1965.

In making these arguments, this chapter emphasizes the significance of Filipino migration in the interrelated U.S. immigration and Asian American historiographical discourses about the mid–twentieth century, debates that have focused mainly on Japanese American relocation and internment during World War II, restrictive immigration legislation codified in the McCarran-Walter Act, and the repeal of Chinese exclusion. Finally, this chapter contributes to the growing historical and sociological literature on the racialized, gendered, and classed recruitment of laborers from outside of the United States during this period, most notably Mexican American *braceros* and Filipino Navy men, in the hope that future comparative study will be conducted on these marginalized groups in U.S. immigration history.

A DYNAMIC MEASURE

The mass migration of Filipino exchange nurses to the United States was an unintended, though historically significant, outcome of U.S. cold war agendas and post–World War II labor shortages. In 1948, the American government through the U.S. Information and Education Act established the EVP. The general objective of the program was to promote a better understanding of the United States in other countries. However, the motivations for establishing the program were rooted in cold war politics. According to Senate reports, "Hostile propaganda campaigns directed against democracy, human welfare, freedom, truth, and the United States, spearheaded by the Government of the Soviet Union and the Communist Parties throughout the world," called for "dynamic measures to disseminate truth."[2] One of the "dynamic measures" that the Senate proposed was an educational exchange service that would involve the interchange of persons, knowledge, and skills.

EVP participants from abroad engaged in both work and study in their sponsoring U.S. institutions, for which they received a monthly stipend. Although the Senate discussions of the exchange program did not refer to the U.S. health care system specifically, several thousand U.S. agencies and institutions were able to sponsor exchange participants, including the American Nurses Association (ANA) and individual hospitals. The U.S. government issued exchange visitor visas for a maximum stay of two years. Upon the completion of the program, the U.S. and the sending countries' governments expected the exchange participants to return to their country of origin.

The Philippines and Filipino nurses were not the sole participants of the EVP. U.S. institutions sponsored exchange visitors from countries in Europe as well as Asia. The occupational background of exchange participants also varied. Furthermore, American nurses also participated in the program, as exchange visitor nurses in foreign countries. The International Unit of the ANA, in cooperation with the International Council of Nurses, assisted American nurses with exchange placements abroad as well as foreign nurses with exchange placements in the United States.

Although the EVP did not specify particular migration flows, in the 1950s the international migrations of exchange nurses (both to non-U.S. countries as well as to the United States) were highly unequal, with exchanges between the United States and northern Europe dominating the arrangements made by the ANA. From 1957 to 1959, the ANA arranged first-time exchange placements for seventy-six American nurses; over half of these nurses visited Great Britain and Denmark, and the others primarily visited other northern European countries: France, Sweden, Germany, Switzerland, Holland, Norway, Finland, and Scotland.[3] Throughout the 1950s, ANA arrangements for foreign exchange nurses in the United States mirrored these itineraries with Danish, Swedish, and British exchange nurses numerically dominating those from other countries, including the Philippines.[4]

However, once Filipino nurses and the Philippine government became actively involved in the EVP, the Philippines began to dominate participation in the program.[5] According to Purita Asperilla, by the late 1960s, 80 percent of exchange participants in the United States were from the Philippines, with nurses comprising the majority of Filipino exchange visitors. The EVP facilitated the first wave of mass migration of Filipino nurses abroad: between 1956 and 1969, over eleven thousand Filipino nurses participated in the program.[6] The increasing numbers of Filipino exchange nurses would begin the profound transformation of the racial and ethnic composition of foreign-trained nurses in the United States. According to Tomoji Ishi, by the late 1960s, nurses from the Philippines comprised the overwhelming majority of exchange visitor nurses in the United States.[7]

While these exchange nurse migrant flows prefigured some of the racialized, classed, and gendered dynamics of post-1965 migration, aspects of the EVP also reconstructed and perpetuated U.S. colonial agendas that had been institutionalized in early twentieth-century scholarship programs to the United States, such as the pensionado program and Rockefeller scholarship programs. It recreated a type of sojourner, elite class of Filipino professionals who would study in the United States for a limited period, earn U.S. educational credentials and gain U.S. work experience, and eventually return to work in the Philippines after having been exposed to U.S. professional trends. In doing so, the EVP also recreated the racialized social, cultural, and intellectual hierarchies of U.S. colonialism in which U.S. institutions — medical, political, educational — were superior to those of the Philippines. Like previous U.S. colonial programs, it perpetuated this hierarchy through the U.S. sponsorship and training of foreign students in which women, specifically nurses, played a unique role. As one U.S. nursing study of exchange visitor nurses proposed, "What better persons can communicate our achievements to other countries than the nurse with her high code of ethics? What better ambassador can we expect to have? The nurse belongs to an honorable, dignified profession. It is she, who on her return home will mingle both with the average and the influential people of her country. She will tell them about the way of life in the United States."[8]

The term "ambassador" usually refers to a representative from the "home" country in a foreign territory; American nurses' assumptions that U.S. training could transform a foreign exchange nurse into an even better "ambassador" for the United States illustrated the complex intersections among the international, transnational, and national dynamics of professional nursing training. The study outlined the ways an international exchange program could simultaneously override traditional national boundaries while at the same time reinscribing U.S. nationalist agendas. American nursing leaders expected the foreign exchange nurse to learn about the national nursing achievements of the United States and to then disseminate this chauvinism on her return home.

If the EVP recreated colonial inequalities, why did thousands of Filipino nurses participate in the program? The racialized hierarchies shaped by U.S. colonialism in the Philippines help explain this phenomenon. Filipino nurses were attracted to the prestige attached to studying and working in the United States, a prestige partly informed by the complex intersecting outcomes of Spanish and U.S. colonialism in the archipelago that had bestowed a unique form of socioeconomic mobility to those few Filipinos who had received professional training abroad. While these outcomes undoubtedly predisposed Filipino professionals to work and study abroad, Filipino nurses themselves contributed to the perpetuation of this prestige, perhaps in the belief that their experience abroad carved an international avenue of recognition and authority for themselves. For example, the FNA perpetuated the idealization of American work and educational experience through news stories in the *Philip-*

pine Journal of Nursing (*PJN*). Simply participating in the EVP was newsworthy. In 1960, the *PJN* published each of the names and alma maters of the more than one hundred Filipino exchange nurses leaving for the United States every two to three months.[9] It also featured Filipino nurses in the United States for the professional recognition they had obtained abroad. When Chicago's American Hospital honored Juanita Jimenez, a Filipino nurse participant in its Industrial Trainee Program, as "Best Nurse of the Year," the *PJN* featured Jimenez as "a silver lining in our profession."[10]

Related to the prestige of study and work abroad was the opportunity afforded these professional sojourners to personally transform themselves through travel. In their advertisements, Philippine travel agencies (which also functioned as recruitment and placement agencies for Filipino exchange nurses in the United States) emphasized the transformative potential of travel that nursing work overseas could provide. The rhetoric of these advertisements ironically echoed the early twentieth-century recruitment of American nurses to the Philippine colony. If travel could transform American nurses into cosmopolitan, modern women through the visual and experiential consumption of exotic places outside of the United States in the early twentieth century, so too could it transform Filipino women working as nurses outside of the Philippines in the mid–twentieth century. Travel agency placement perks for Filipino exchange nurses included free hotel accommodations in Hong Kong and Tokyo and a sightseeing stopover in Honolulu.[11] Such travel through working abroad was like a personal makeover. As one travel agency advertisement in the *PJN* targeted Filipino nurses: "Visit those far-away castles, climb those dazzling mountains, taste exotic foods and indulge in fabulous shopping bargains. . . . And like a dream, you can fly to all those interesting places, meet interesting people, and *come back, a more interesting you!*"[12]

The poor working conditions of nurses in the Philippines in the mid–twentieth century added to the prestige and transformative potential attached to work and study in the United States. Filipino nurses' dissatisfaction with their work schedules, opportunities, and salaries in the Philippines motivated them to go abroad and take a chance on a new work environment. For example, Milagros Rabara applied for an exchange placement to avoid an evening work shift. She explained, "The place I was working in as an industrial nurse, they tried to change my time and I didn't like it, my schedule time. . . . I used to work in the morning and then they let me work in the evening, which was very difficult for me to go home. I had to take a bus, maybe a ride of an hour. . . . So I left the company and I said, Let me go around and see what I can do. And I found this agency and they said we have an [exchange] opening for November."[13]

The limited number of days off at her hospital in the Philippines motivated Lourdes Velasco to apply to the exchange program. She recalled, "We heard that here [in the United States] you're off two days a week. . . . We were off [in the Philippines] only two days a month. In 1963, after graduation, one of my close relatives was getting married. I could not attend the wedding because I did not have the day off. I missed that important wedding."[14]

Favoritism on the job alienated Filipino nurses who had worked in their communities for many years. After Hermila Rabe graduated with a University of Santo Tomas nursing degree in 1954, she worked at a hospital in Tarlac, which was located one hour from her hometown, for twelve and a half years. Mila (as she preferred to be called) claimed that she "got the best training in the world" in Tarlac: "I was [a] staff nurse. I was assigned to every department." Although her father initially objected to her decision to go to the United States as an exchange visitor, Rabe eventually used the program to leave the Philippines in 1967. She explained, "I was so disgusted with the director of the hospital. . . . There was favoritism. I am supposed to be one of the candidates of the chief nurse at [the] hospital, but there is another nurse who is junior, my junior at the University of Santo Tomas. I graduated in 1954, and she graduated in 1955. But she is with that director. I don't like that and I don't want to be like that. . . . My father was so afraid to let me go here. But I discussed with him about [the] hospital, that they are not treating us equally. So I convinced my father."[15]

Filipino nurses working in the Philippines also suffered from low wages and little professional respect. Some government agencies employing nurses paid them lower wages than their janitors, drivers, and messengers. In the mid-1960s, Filipino nurses earned approximately 200 to 300 pesos monthly for working six days a week, including holidays and overtime if necessary.[16] These low nursing salaries contributed to their desire to go abroad to countries like the United States where, in the mid-1960s, general duty nurses earned approximately $400 to $500 per month.[17] Even if Filipino exchange nurses earned a fraction of U.S. nursing salaries with their stipends, the amount was often greater than their salary in the Philippines.

Filipino nurses also took the opportunity to go abroad because professional and financial opportunities materialized for some Filipino exchange nurses in the United States. Contradictory narratives about the program emerged from my interviews. Some former exchange nurses harshly criticized the educational component of their exchange placements as inadequate; others believed that the program successfully promoted professional and cultural exchange. Luz Alerta, an exchange nurse at the University of Texas, Galveston, from 1967 to 1969, related, "[The EVP] was good because you go through orientation and then . . . you have sightseeing in the community, and then . . . you are brought to the mayor's office. It's a small town, so you go to the stores and they give you gifts. . . . Most of the people in Galveston are Baptists, so we are invited by the church. . . . They invite us for salads on some evenings. . . . I think it's very good."[18]

Some exchange nurses characterized their work duties as exploitation; others found these experiences rewarding. Josephine Abalos praised the collaboration between the exchange nurses and medical students during her exchange visit at the University of Pennsylvania, an interaction that the first Filipino nursing students under U.S. colonial rule had also interpreted as exciting and prestigious. Jo (as she preferred to be called) recollected that "it was fun working with medical students, too, and exchanging ideas."[19] Ofelia Boado also reminisced fondly about her exchange visit at the Children's Hospital in Washington, D.C.: "I liked it very, very much. All children, no adults. . . . We had asthma. We had overdose of aspirin. We had, they call it, wringer injury, when children put their hands in the washing machine. . . . The work was rewarding, very rewarding."[20]

Although some Filipino exchange nurses acknowledged that the stipends they received were minimal, they still interpreted their economic situation positively. Ofelia Boado admitted that "the pay was not so good. But in 1963 the milk was, like, 21 cents and everything was cheap. We were paying just $95 for an apartment in Philadelphia. . . . It was good for what we get in payment."[21] In addition to wage differentials between nurses working in the Philippines and in the United States, the devaluation of the Philippine peso exponentially increased the earning power of Filipino nurses working in America. The devaluation began in 1946 with the Tydings Rehabilitation Act, which provided much-needed economic aid to a devastated post–World War II Philippine economy, yet at the same time established the exchange rate of the peso–dollar at two to one. This economic disparity would increase over time. By 1971, 1 U.S. dollar was equivalent to 6.25 Philippine pesos. A Filipino working as a staff nurse in a New York hospital earned a minimum of 60,000 pesos annually given this exchange rate. In the Philippines, the Filipino nurse earned an annual salary of approximately 4,200 pesos. In other words, a Filipino nurse working in the Philippines needed to work twelve years to earn what she could make as a nurse in the United States in one year.[22] As Boado observed, "The pay [in the United States] was good compared to what I was getting in the Philippines. . . . It became so clear to me that many nurses come here not for advancement but for pay, for really good pay."[23] Given this neocolonial economic disparity, some Filipino exchange nurses manipulated the exchange visitor program to serve their own agendas, for example, by working sixteen-hour shifts to earn more money.

However, the motivations of Filipino nurses for participating in the EVP went beyond simple monetary calculations. Filipino exchange nurses acted on the transformative potential of experience abroad by augmenting their socioeconomic status through the accumulation of material goods unobtainable and new forms of leisure unavailable in the Philippines. Their stipends in U.S. dollars, combined with the availability of credit cards and layaway plans, enabled Filipino exchange nurses to purchase stereos, kitchen appliances, and cosmetics unobtainable to all except the affluent elite in the Philippines. They engaged in forms of leisure completely unavailable in the Philippines: Broadway shows, Lincoln Center performances, travel within the United States. They lived in their own apartment and stayed out late at night. As Boado recalled, "You're very independent. You have your own apartment. In the Philippines, you live in the dorm, where everything closes at 9 o'clock P.M. Or, even if you stay at home, you don't go home late in the night or anything like that."[24]

The new "independence" of Filipino exchange nurses, however, did not translate into assimilation in the United States or separation from the Philippines. While the program created opportunities to escape family surveillance and discipline for some exchange nurses, the parents of Filipino nurses also used the exchange program to increase their surveillance and discipline. After graduating from the University of Santo Tomas in 1953, Ofelia Boado worked at San Juan de Dios Hospital in Manila, which she described as "a beautiful hospital." She worked at that hospital for almost twelve years before coming to the United States as an exchange nurse in 1964. According to Boado, she was uninterested in going abroad because she was content with her work in the Philippines: "I was satisfied with what I was doing out there. . . . I wasn't prepared for [going abroad to the United States]. Some of my classmates were here and they were doing great, but that didn't really attract me." She made plans to go abroad at the request of her father, who wanted her to visit her younger sister in Massachusetts, meet her sister's new boyfriend, and confirm that the boyfriend was a decent man. In Boado's case, the opportunity to go abroad through the EVP facilitated a type of substitute parental surveillance over a Filipino daughter already abroad. She explained:

> Then my sister . . . maybe four or five years younger than me, she graduated [with a degree in] chemistry, and she wanted to come over to the United States. So she came over. And then while she was here at Massachusetts General Hospital, she fell in love with a guy. This was the truth I'm telling you. She fell in love with a guy who was working with her in Mass. General. And then my father, being strict—you know how fathers are—he told me, "Why don't you go out there and check your sister? Check the man." So I said, "Why am I going to the United States without work? What will I do there?" So I applied . . . as an exchange visitor. . . . So I came here. I found nothing wrong with Chester, [who is now] my brother-in-law . . . nothing wrong with him. So I wrote back to my father. In fact, they are married for thirty years now, you see.[25]

Julieta Luistro's exchange visitor experience illustrated one way that Filipino mothers as well as fathers used the exchange program to discipline their nurse-daughters. Soon after Luistro's graduation from St. Paul's College in Manila in 1964, she left the Philippines under the auspices of the EVP. According to Luistro, her mother had arranged the exchange placement for her to temporarily separate her from her boyfriend in the Philippines: "My mother arranged [my exchange placement]. She knew this travel agent, a friend of the family, who recruits nurses to go to the States. So she arranged for me to join a group to go to Michigan. She did it on her own. I wasn't that ready to come to the

States because I had a boyfriend. . . . So that, I guess, that's one way to keep us apart so I won't get married right away after graduation."[26]

These stories speak to the diversity of Filipino exchange nurses' reasons for going abroad, but in general, Filipino parents encouraged and supported their nurse-daughters to go abroad because professional work and advanced study in the United States, and specifically *outside* the Philippines, enabled Filipino nurses to enhance their own and their family's class status *within* the Philippines. By the time of Philippine independence in 1946, one way the Philippine landholding, agricultural elite solidified its social status was by sending its sons and daughters abroad for training as doctors, lawyers, and other white-collar professionals.[27] Although they were unable to transform their family into this landholding, agricultural elite in the Philippines, one way Filipino exchange nurses in the United States enhanced their family's socioeconomic status was by sending material goods (gifts known as *pasalubongs*) to their family and friends back home. The popularization of these transnational material exchanges led to the creation of *balikbayan* boxes manufactured by Filipino American entrepreneurs in the 1980s to specifically ship these pasalubongs back to the Philippines. Vicente Rafael has astutely observed that "such boxes are the material evidence of immigrant success as much as they are of the promise of immigration itself. Thus they do constitute the materialization of a desire realizable only outside the nation, yet recognizable only within its borders."[28]

The material evidence of exchange visitor "success" (also realized only outside, but recognized only inside the Philippines) preceded and helped shape the contours of this notion of Filipino immigrant success in the post-1965 period. Thus, despite her separation from her boyfriend, Julieta Luistro welcomed the opportunity to go to the United States as an exchange nurse because it enabled her to fulfill this particular desire. She observed that other Filipino nurses abroad purchased American goods and sent them back to their friends and family members in the Philippines, and she longed for the kind of achievement embodied in this material exchange: "I had a classmate in high school who already was a nurse and here in the States at the time. . . . My cousin was in Kentucky at that time . . . and she was sending Avon cosmetics to me. . . . And my classmate was sending me Avon cosmetics also. . . . They have products here that we don't have in the Philippines. And that, I guess, I sort of would want that to happen to me too, to be able to send things to my mom at home when I get here. And that's what I did."[29] Such success motivated other Filipino families to aggressively invest in the travel costs for their nurse-daughter to go abroad. Milagros Rabara related that her family helped pay for her trip to America: "It was Mom's retirement pay I think. It was 3,000. . . . She was taking it from the shoe box."[30]

Filipino exchange nurses' ability to enhance their status in the Philippines helped change their perceptions of themselves. Being in a different country and among new networks of colleagues and friends enabled them to imagine themselves as something other than a Filipino of lower-class or upper-class status in the Philippines, and to become aware of their belonging to a new class of Filipino professionals in the United States. As Josephine Abalos explained, "See, in the Philippines, if you were rich, you were rich. If you were poor, you were poor. Here [in the United States], it equalizes everybody. The work and the salary equalizes. Your status becomes lost. . . . So you were somebody in the Philippines? Too bad. You are somebody here, but everybody else is somebody too, see?"[31]

The prestige and transformative potential of work abroad changed the culture of Philippine nursing training by encouraging not only thousands of other Filipino nurses to go to the United States, but also other young Filipino women to enter nursing school in the hopes of going abroad. In 1962 there were more student applicants for nursing studies than Philippine colleges and schools of nursing were able to accommodate.[32] And going abroad after the study of nursing figured prominently in their plans. In 1963, the president of the FNA asked prospective nursing students why they chose that field of study. She reported, "This may surprise you but about 80% of those asked have answered me that it is because they want to go to the United States and other countries."[33]

Opportunities specifically through the EVP motivated young Filipino women to take up nursing. In the early 1960s, nursing applicants to St. Luke's Hospital School of Nursing in Quezon City, Metro Manila, highlighted opportunities through the program in their statements of purpose.[34] As one graduating member of the class of 1965 wrote in her application, "Many say that nurses have more opportunities to go to the U.S. under the Exchange program. . . . After finishing my nursing course I am planning . . . to go to the United States to specialize in surgical nursing." In another application, a graduating member of the class of 1967 wrote that "the profession offers a wide field of employment especially abroad, through the EVP. . . . After a few years of practice, I would like to go abroad through the EVP."

These young women's applications reflected the popularization of the folklore about America as a land of promise, a folklore first created during the early U.S. colonial period. Through their letters to nursing friends back in the Philippines, Filipino exchange nurses refashioned and perpetuated this folklore as they told stories of high salaries, liberal working policies, and "good living" in the United States.[35] Luz Alerta attributed her decision to become an exchange nurse to the presence of friends and classmates already in the United States who wrote to her. As Milagros Rabara explained, "Most of my classmates were already here in the U.S.A., so I wanted to come."[36] Going abroad became a trend among Filipino nurses. One study revealed that between 1952 and 1965 an average of slightly more than 50 percent of 377 graduates from the University of the Philippines College of Nursing went abroad.[37] However, on their arrival in the United States, the exploitation of Filipino exchange nurses by Philippine recruitment agencies and U.S. sponsoring hospitals challenged romanticized narratives about America.

SIMPLE ARRANGEMENTS, COMPLEX ADJUSTMENTS

Filipino nurses were able to obtain exchange visitor sponsorship from the American Nurses Association and individual U.S. hospitals. The FNA collaborated with the ANA to screen exchange nurses from the Philippines and to process their placement in the United States. Philippine travel agencies worked with U.S. sponsoring hospital administrators to facilitate the placement of Filipino exchange nurses in their institutions.

In editorials in the *PJN,* the FNA boasted about the positive experiences of the nurses they had sponsored in contrast to those nurses who had been placed by travel agencies.[38] Yet, despite these success stories of FNA- and ANA-sponsorship, the overwhelming majority of Filipino exchange nurses bypassed these arrangements partly because the FNA's internal problems had alienated current members and younger Filipino nurses.[39] In the 1950s and early 1960s, interrelated problems of internal power struggles, election fraud, illegal constitution use, and low membership marked a tumultuous period for the FNA. Some members contended that these controversies were aberrations; however, one article in the *PJN* strongly criticized the FNA and expressed ambivalence about the future of the professional organization: "I wonder if our leaders realized the effect of their attitude to the younger nurses who are watching their every action! . . . Really the situation is disgusting and discouraging but not altogether hopeless."[40] A group of recent nursing graduates echoed these sentiments: "For once let us go back to our senses. . . . I hope we can now walk again like real professionals among other colleagues."[41]

In contrast to the chaotic nature of the FNA, travel agencies offered potential Filipino exchange nurses "special service" and "simple arrangements." Travel agents working with American sponsoring hospitals targeted Filipino nurses with enticing advertisements in the *PJN*. In 1964, an advertisement for PAL (Philippine Airlines) featured a photograph of a Filipino nurse with the caption, "Training abroad?" The advertisement continued: "Free placement service: PAL will assist you with the choice of a U.S. hospital. You get complete information on employment requirements, terms, living expenses, wardrobe, etc. This is a special service extended by PAL to U.S.-bound Filipino doctors and nurses." In the 1960s, Pan American and Northwest Airlines also targeted the growing numbers of Filipino nurses traveling to the United States as exchange visitors. As one Northwest Airlines advertisement in 1969 beckoned: "189.40 pesos is all the cash you need to fly to the USA on Northwest Orient's 'Fly Now — Pay Later' plan. The balance may be paid in as many as 24 monthly installments. The arrangements are simple."[42]

The speed and efficiency of travel agency-arranged exchange placements attracted Filipino nurses. Lourdes Velasco characterized obtaining an exchange placement as an "easy" process because, as she explained, "We had a travel agent. It facilitates [the application]. I don't think there's anyone I knew who did not have a travel agent."[43] Although travel agents arranged exchange placements for qualified nursing candidates such as Velasco, who had a baccalaureate nursing degree from St. Paul's College, the speed of their arrangements at times resulted in the placement of unqualified exchange nurses. In 1963, the FNA reported that they had discovered one exchange nurse with the necessary paperwork to leave the Philippines who was not a registered nurse.[44]

Travel agencies expedited exchange placements because they profited from the airplane tickets purchased by Filipino nurses going abroad and particularly from the payment plans for these tickets, popularly known as "Fly Now, Pay Later" plans. Many Philippine travel agencies offered these plans, in which the nurse placed a down payment of 10 percent of the airfare and paid the balance over the following months through salary deductions. While these plans allowed nurses to purchase an airplane ticket with an initial minimal amount, they charged an exorbitantly high interest rate for the remaining balance. In 1966, one agency advertised a 12 percent annual interest rate for the balance of the airfare.[45]

Upon arrival in the United States, hospital exploitation challenged the romanticized folklore about America as a land of promise, and about the EVP as a mutually beneficial program for the exchangees as well as their U.S. sponsoring institutions. Travel agencies may have expedited the placement process to sign on as many Filipino nurses as possible on their Fly Now, Pay Later plans, but they had little interest in the quality of work conditions and educational programs of sponsoring hospitals in the United States. Many Filipino nurses placed by travel agencies encountered discriminatory work conditions and inadequate orientation programs at their sponsoring hospitals.[46]

Some U.S. hospital administrators offered little, if any, assistance to new Filipino exchange nurses while they adjusted to living in a new environment, leaving them to fend for themselves. After finishing her one-year exchange placement at the University of Pennsylvania, Jo Abalos began a new placement at an inner-city hospital in Chicago. She recalled, "Nobody met us at the airport. There were only two of us, so we took a cab from the airport and arrived [at the hospital] about 4 in the morning."[47]

Sponsoring hospitals also varied their exchange nurse policies and orientation programs over time. Although the University of Pennsylvania arranged dormitory housing for Abalos during her exchange placement in 1961, it did not provide any housing arrangements for Christina Hing during her placement in 1962. Hing related that in the Philippines even professional nurses resided in a hospital dormitory. In Pennsylvania, she had to find her own housing accommodations without her sponsor's assistance: "Once here I had to buy groceries, cook, everything." She characterized the beginning of her exchange visitor experience as "real culture shock."[48]

Even when sponsoring hospitals attempted to provide temporary lodging for newly arrived exchange visitors, at times these provisions were poorly planned. In 1964, Fortunata Kennedy arrived in the United States with fifteen other exchange nurses. A representative of the Chicago hospital that sponsored them met them at the airport and accompanied them to a YMCA. Fortune (as she preferred to be called) recollected, "When we got there, the clerk denied ever receiving reservations for us. We ended up with three nurses sharing one small room. The next day, one of the nurses was able to contact a friend who had been in Chicago for over a year. Through her, we were able to find a place to stay. No one really helped us settle in the U.S. Our initiative and determination made us survive the first few difficult years."[49]

The guidance, support, and company of other Filipino exchange nurses facilitated their adjustment to the United States and helped make exchange visits enjoyable even in the midst of hospital abandonment, exploitation, and discrimination. For example, Ofelia Boado and a nurse-friend, a colleague at San Juan de Dios Hospital, arrived as exchange visitors in the United States at the same time. According to Boado, they traveled to New York City during some weekends and visited other nurse-friends from the Philippines who were working there. Julieta Luistro arrived in Michigan as part of a group of five Filipino exchange nurses. They shared a house subsidized by the sponsoring hospital and helped each other settle into their new environment.

However, while the EVP facilitated the reunion of nurse-friends and the start of new friendships in the United States, it also separated Filipino nurse-friends in the Philippines. Lourdes Velasco and a nurse-friend planned to go abroad together as exchange nurses. According to Velasco, the company of her friend motivated her to apply to the program only one year after graduation: "She's the reason why I wanted to leave right away. Because we were best friends. . . . We became classmates. So we were close." However, her best friend was unable to go abroad because of a medical condition. Velasco lamented, "I was so unhappy because she could not come because [of] her X-ray. All our plans the two of us were planning: 'Oh, this is how we will live there. We will attend all the cultural [events]. We'll come to New York. We'll do this. We'll do that.' And she could not come. . . . I found out at the last minute that she could not join us. She was so disappointed."[50] After Velasco left for the United States, she lost contact with her best friend. She said that she was still trying to locate her whereabouts.

Aside from providing inadequate settlement assistance, some U.S. hospital administrators abused the educational component of the EVP by assigning exchange nurses the work of nurse's aides.[51] Other hospitals did not offer any orientations or educational programs. As Josephine Abalos explained, "To be a hospital accepted in the Exchange Visitor Program, you were supposed to give training to these foreign grad nurses to enhance their previous education. . . . But a lot of us didn't have any orientation. They just said, 'Look, this is the med-surg unit. We have eighteen patients here. They're all yours. Okay?' That's the kind of orientation."[52]

Many sponsoring hospitals used exchange nurses as an inexpensive labor supply to alleviate growing nursing shortages in the post–World War II period.[53] In 1961, the ANA conducted a spot check of nonfederal general hospitals and found that the need for general duty nurses was particularly significant; 23 percent of these positions were vacant. Some American hospital administrators took advantage of the *exchange* status of these nurses by assigning them the work of registered nurses and then compensating them with a minimal stipend. U.S. taxes further reduced the stipend. Christina Hing related that in 1962 she earned $46.50 per week as an exchange nurse in a Philadelphia hospital. According to ANA statistics, the general duty nurse in a Philadelphia nongovernmental hospital in 1960 earned a weekly average of $71.50.[54] Using these examples, a sponsoring hospital could exploit the exchange nurse by having her perform general nursing duties and then compensating her with a fraction (approximately two-thirds) of a general duty nurse's average salary.

Filipino exchange nurses were not passive victims of hospital mistreatment. They organized themselves to improve their work conditions. For example, in 1967, a group of forty Filipino exchange nurses filed a libel suit against their sponsoring hospital, St. Barnabus Hospital in New Jersey, after the hospital dismissed nine Filipino exchange nurses who were accused of stealing hospital property.[55] The group considered the dismissal excessive and characterized the accusation as an affront to their integrity. Before the suit took place, the hospital reinstated the dismissed nurses. The group of nurses and the hospital then reached a compromise that included the withdrawal of the libel suit and the resignation of the hospital's coordinator and supervisor of exchange visitors.

In 1967, Filipino exchange nurses in Galveston, Texas established a Galveston chapter of the Philippine Nurses Association (PNA; leaders of the Filipino Nurses Association had renamed the professional nursing organization in 1966).[56] Members organized social events, such as a welcome party and beach party, for new groups of Filipino exchange nurses at their hospital. They also petitioned their hospital for an increase in pay, the right to transfer to another hospital department after one year, and an extension of cooking privileges in their dormitory. At least one of their requests, the increase in pay, was successful.

The activities of the PNA-Galveston chapter illustrate the way Filipino nurses in the United States simultaneously relied on Filipino professional cultural traditions while they created new ones. In 1965, Yolanda Fabros wrote to the FNA secretary soliciting advice on how to organize a chapter of the professional organization among the group of Filipino exchange nurses in Galveston. According to Fabros, the group wanted to organize "as a part of our mother organization" and to "be recognized as one chapter in this part of the United States."[57] Fabros's letter revealed that Filipino exchange nurses in the United States longed for professional membership in the Philippines. Yet, instead of simply joining the FNA on an individual basis, these nurses wanted to be recognized as a chapter abroad.

The formation of the PNA-Galveston chapter also reflected the complex interaction between international nursing programs and nurses' nationalist yearnings. Although one objective of the EVP was to increase understanding of the United States in other countries, the negative experiences of Filipino exchange nurses in the United States motivated them to learn more about the professional nursing association of the Philippines. The program inadvertently inspired interaction between Filipino exchange nurses in Galveston and the PNA, interactions that might not have occurred in the Philippines, where the association suffered from tumultuous internal divisions.

Although American as well as Filipino nurses critiqued sponsoring hospitals' exploitation of exchange nurses, several factors hindered their development of a transnational professional consciousness and solidarity. Filipino exchange nurses turned to each other and to the PNA because they observed the ways American nursing supervisors took advantage of their labor. Some supervisors exploited exchange nurses by assigning them to work in the least desirable areas of the hospital and on the least desirable work shifts, knowing that the exchange nurse's visa status depended on her sponsorship from the hospital. Luzviminda Micabalo also observed that they would change exchange nurses' work schedules suddenly, whenever they deemed necessary: "I thought they were exploiting the foreign nurses . . . in the way they scheduled work. It wasn't fair . . . they would schedule nurses to work in the morning, and then they would change your schedule without appropriate notice and shift you to night shift. Or you would be working night shift and if they needed somebody to work in the morning shift or afternoon shift, they would change it."[58] Filipino nurses further criticized nursing supervisors for offering American nurses better working conditions and schedules at their expense. In Purificacion Capulong's study of Filipino exchange nurses, several of them complain that "the Filipino nurses always get the 'dirty' job" and that supervisors gave American nurses their choice of assignments, while they were "doing night duty for three months" or "evening duty for six months."[59]

Furthermore, although the ANA also criticized abuses of the EVP, they did so in very different ways. In 1960, the ANA published a statement expressing its concern over the abuses of the program.[60] The ANA lamented that these abuses, such as misleading advertisements, which featured the educational components of the program at U.S. hospitals that later did not provide them, created disappointment and frustration for the foreign nurses. However, it also interpreted hospitals' exploitation of exchange nurses as detrimental to American nurses because, the ANA believed, the low stipends of exchange nurses lowered the economic status of American nurses. The ANA harshly criticized the use of exchange nurses to fulfill the duties of American registered nurses because exchange nurses were not licensed according to U.S. professional standards. They argued that this practice jeopardized patients' safety. Thus, the ANA's major concerns focused on the professional status of American nurses and the welfare of American patients, who were administered care by a growing number of Filipino exchange nurses. As I discuss in Chapter 6, the divisive effect of such rhetoric, which pitted American nurses against Filipino nurses, foreshadowed the divisions between American professional nursing organizations and Filipino nurses' organizations in the United States in the 1970s and 1980s, when U.S. hospitals increased their use of foreign-trained nurses, the majority of whom were Filipino.

By the mid-1960s, the use of Filipino exchange nurses as employees appeared to be the rule rather than the exception. A study committee of the Philippine Department of Labor characterized the EVP as "a handy recruitment device" and "a loophole for the circumvention of United States immigration laws."[61] And some Filipino exchange nurses themselves were well aware of this. According to Priscilla Santayana, "[The

Exchange Visitor Program] was work. The 'exchange' was a misnomer. When you came here, you were working as a staff nurse with a stipend. They didn't call it salary because if they call it a salary that means you are a permanent employee. . . . Everybody knew that."[62]

According to some Philippine reports, there were few, if any, redeeming qualities about the program. In 1966, Philippine Congress member Epifanio Castillejos visited the United States to survey the situation of Filipino exchange nurses and severely criticized the program: "Almost every Filipino nurse I met had problems which ran the gamut from discrimination in stipend, as well as in the nature and amount of work they are made to do, to the lack of in-service or specialized training in the hospitals they work in. . . . I have seen with my own eyes the extent and the seriousness of their helplessness and hopelessness."[63]

One might surmise that such reports of discrimination and exploitation would discourage further migration to the United States through the EVP, but Lourdes Velasco's story reveals the opposite. She arrived in the United States in 1964, after negative reports of the program had already been publicized. According to Velasco, she and her best friend were in "a rush to apply" to the program.[64] They were certainly not the only ones. Over three thousand Filipino nurses participated in the program between 1967 and 1970, after Castillejos declared that the situation of Filipino exchange nurses was one of helplessness and hopelessness.[65]

The persistence of Filipino nurses' participation in the EVP suggests that, although reports of hospital exploitation, inadequate educational programs, and minimal stipends in the United States may have compelled some nurses to rethink their idealization of the program, the ability of Filipino exchange nurses to transform their socioeconomic status continued to attract subsequent generations of nurse graduates to work abroad. By the early 1960s, Filipino exchange nurses continued to manipulate the program to serve their own agendas, not only by trying to earn as much money as possible, but by remaining in the United States indefinitely.

In 1960, FNA President Luisa Alvarez reported that many Filipino exchange nurses in Chicago complained about the relatively short length of their visit. According to these nurses, the two-year period was insufficient time to reap "the benefits of the program."[66] They inquired if it were possible to extend their visit to a period of three to five years. When extensions did not materialize, some nurses returned to the Philippines after their two-year stay. However, others attempted to bypass the foreign residency requirement altogether and to change their visa status while they were still in the United States.

Although the U.S. Mutual Educational and Cultural Exchange Act of 1961 mandated that exchange visitors return to their country of origin or another foreign country for a period of two years before applying for a U.S. immigrant visa, Filipino exchange nurses employed multiple strategies to avoid returning to the Philippines. Some married American citizens; others immigrated to Canada; some exited the United States through Canada or Mexico and then reentered as students; still others used a combination of requests by American universities, the Philippine Consul General, and American hospital employers to petition the Exchange Visitor Waiver Board of the Department of Health, Education, and Welfare for a waiver of the foreign residence requirement.

When these strategies failed and the Immigration and Naturalization Service set their date for departure, some Filipino exchange nurses brought their case to the U.S. Court of Appeals in an attempt to overturn INS rulings. In November 1967, the U.S. Court of Appeals heard petitions from two exchange nurses who had avoided returning to the Philippines by temporarily relocating to Canada.[67] Lilia Velasco entered the United States as an exchange nurse in 1961. When her exchange status expired in 1963, she immigrated to Canada and then reentered the United States several times as a temporary visitor. In 1966, the INS determined that Velasco's residence in Canada subverted the purpose and intent of the exchange program. Although the INS directed her to depart from the United States, it also informed her that a hospital employer could apply for a waiver of her foreign residence requirement. Two American hospitals, the Kaiser Foundation Hospital in Los Angeles and the Roosevelt Hospital in Chicago, applied for such a waiver on her behalf. However, the Exchange Visitor Waiver Review Board denied the waiver.

Filipino exchange nurse Nellie Morales faced a similar situation. She had entered the United States as an exchange visitor in 1961 and returned to the Philippines in early 1964 after the expiration of her exchange visa. However, after a stay of only six weeks, she immigrated to Canada. In December 1965, Morales reentered the United States from Canada as a nonimmigrant visitor and received a U.S. immigrant visa in January 1966. The INS requested the Department of State to determine whether Morales satisfied the foreign residence requirements of the exchange program. When the Department of State reported that Morales had not complied with the requirements, the INS advised her to depart the United States by September 16, 1966. Chicago's Roosevelt Hospital filed a petition for waiver of Morales's foreign residence requirement, but the Exchange Visitor Waiver Review Board denied the waiver.

Velasco and Morales petitioned the U.S. Court of Appeals to review the INS rulings for their deportations, but the court sided with the INS and dismissed their petitions. Interpreting the foreign residence requirement of the exchange program as residence in the visitor's country of origin or, in the case of these Filipino exchange nurses, in an "undeveloped" country, the court ruled that exchange visitors "should return to their native countries to practice their professions and skills, or to do so in undeveloped countries. It would seem obvious Canada would not come under such a classification."[68] Although the court's ruling theoretically applied to all exchange visitors, its insistence that Velasco and Morales return to an "undeveloped" country reveals the U.S. government's understanding and use of global hierarchies in its attempt to control Filipino nurse migrants' mobility.

Despite these rulings, Filipino exchange nurses continued to attempt to subvert control over their mobility in creative ways. One employed a lawyer to argue that hospital employers' exploitation of her labor voided her exchange status, thus freeing her from the exchange visitors' foreign residence requirement. After participating in the EVP at St. Barnabus Medical Center in New Jersey and Columbus Hospital in Chicago from 1965 to 1967, Marina Alonzo claimed that "she was not in fact an Exchange Visitor although she had entered the United States in that capacity." At her INS hearing, Alonzo's counsel offered to prove that her hospital sponsors brought Alonzo to the United States only to relieve a nursing shortage and not to participate in the exchange program. According to Alonzo, "Fraud was practiced upon her in that instead of the anticipated benefits of studying United States techniques in nursing which she could take back to her own country, she was merely put in charge of an abnormally large patient-load and given no training at all." Alonzo petitioned the U.S. Court of Appeals to review the INS ruling of her deportation, but the court responded that "if a fraud occurred, it appears that petitioner was a party to it."[69]

These court cases illustrate one of the striking contradictions of the

EVP: the ways in which the interests of hospital employers and Filipino exchange nurses complemented one another, although the former group exploited the latter as a cheap labor supply. With the same end in mind — having Filipino nurses remain indefinitely in the United States — Filipino nurses and U.S. hospital employers worked together to subvert the immigration restrictions of U.S. government agencies. These court cases also reflected the conflicts among U.S. institutions — in this case, the divergent interests of government agencies and hospitals — regarding the migration and employment of foreign-trained, mainly Filipino, nurses. These conflicts would only escalate over time in the post-1965 period. Meanwhile, across the Pacific Ocean, the complicated alliances between Filipino nurses and their U.S. hospital employers would contribute to the escalating concerns among Philippine government and health officials about the changing desires of Filipino nurses working abroad.

PRIDE AND PREJUDICE

Filipino exchange nurses' desire to remain indefinitely in the United States became a cause of alarm for Philippine government officials and nursing leaders, who interpreted nurses' duties as an integral part of Philippine nation building. Songs such as "The Filipino Nurses' Hymn" promoted this relationship between nursing and Philippine nationalism with lyrics such as: "We pledge . . . to build a better nation that is healthy and great." The hymn conjured images of Filipino nurses "traveling on" to the different regions that comprise the Philippine nation: "In towns and upland terraces/ In plains, in hills and mountains."[70]

Since it had become a trend for new Filipino nurse graduates to go abroad, commencement speeches became one forum for expressing these concerns regarding the relationship between nursing and Philippine nation building. In her commencement speech to the 1966 graduating class of the Philippine General Hospital School of Nursing, Assistant Secretary for Cultural Affairs Pura Castrence characterized exchange nurses' refusal to return to the Philippines as a national problem: "What is relevant is the problem of our nurses' restlessness to go to the United States — and remain there. . . . Why, you wonder, perhaps, has this problem of nurses become almost a national problem? The reason is simple. The country needs you nurses here. There are in the Philippines only 300 rural health units with a full complement of 1 physician, 1 nurse, 1 midwife, and 1 sanitary inspector. . . . there are 112 units without physician or nurse."[71]

Government officials highlighted the presence of disease and suffering in the Philippines in an attempt to link Filipino nurses' duties to national concerns. In his 1965 commencement speech at the Martinez Memorial School of Nursing, former Philippine Secretary of Health Paulino Garcia pleaded with new nurse graduates to serve Filipinos in the Philippines: "Do not even consider the thought of staying abroad permanently. Remember that your people need you, that your country should have first call on your services. . . . As nurses, you are the indispensable ally of the doctors in the never ending fight against disease and death. . . . You can do this, but you must do it here, in our own country and among our own people. You must do it in the rural areas. Thousands of mothers still die in childbirth because they do not receive proper obstetrical care. Thousands of children succumb to diseases the cures for which are known. They would not die if there were nurses around, nurses who can administer injections or give the proper medicines to them."[72] Such rhetoric ironically resembled early twentieth-century U.S. colonial narratives that portrayed the Philippines as a diseased (as well as feminized and infantilized place) in need of rescue. However, although many Philippine health officials had adopted discourses of Western medicine and the belief in its "power to heal," they called on Filipino nurses for such rescue.

Although Philippine government officials spoke about these national concerns with urgency, they tempered their appeals with empathy for the nurses' ambition to go abroad. They too recognized the unique socioeconomic success that Filipino exchange nurses had achieved through work abroad. In his address Garcia admitted, "Do not get me wrong, my dear, dedicated young nurses. I do not blame you for aspiring the way you do, for wishing for yourselves a life of relative ease and comfort."[73] And Castrence acknowledged the limited control they had over nurse migrants' mobility: "You enjoy, of course, from the bill of rights of our Constitution, the right of movement, the right to choose where you want to live and work."[74]

Such acknowledgments produced a sense of helplessness among those who tried to convince Filipino nurses to remain in the Philippines. Garcia presumed that many of these nurse graduates would eventually pursue work abroad: "Go, if you must, to other countries." He pleaded with them only to "give some thought to coming back."[75] Castrence appealed to a nationalistic sense of nursing, but she conceded that the professional definition of nursing signified commitment to all those in the nurse's care, and not primarily to the nurse's countrymen and -women:

> I can offer no solution. I looked over the Florence Nightingale pledge and find nothing that would uphold me in persuading you not to want to serve elsewhere than in your own country. True your pledge says that you are to practice your profession faithfully—does faithfully mean, in your own country, to serve your own suffering fellow-countrymen? True it obliges you to elevate the standards of your profession—does that mean by making sacrifice as the pervasive spirit in your service, and would that mean working for less than you deserve? True it pledges you to a devotion of yourself to the welfare of those committed to your care, but would that signify that you would think of the welfare of your fellow country-men first because that dedication would be the deepening and the broadening of your pledge, which might be its intention? You alone can answer these questions when the time comes, dear nurses.[76]

Yet when the time came for exchange nurses to return to the Philippines, the vast majority who did return planned to go back to the United States.[77] If they shared any new skills they had learned abroad, it was not for very long. They compared salaries, nursing facilities, equipment, and research in the United States with that of the Philippines and became frustrated and disappointed with the latter. These frustrations reflected the ways work abroad had also transformed Filipino exchange nurses' perceptions of their professional training and abilities. Like the Filipino nurses working in San Francisco in the early twentieth century who would not return to the Philippines, much to the chagrin of U.S. colonial officials, mid-twentieth-century Filipino exchange nurses' supposedly temporary work and study in the United States prepared and predisposed them to work in the U.S. health care system, and not in the Philippines. As Josephine Abalos explained, "The thing that I love about American hospitals is that we have enough supplies and equipment. You have catheters. . . . In the Philippines we boiled our own rectal tubes. You use the catheters over and over. . . . Here you just use it once and dump it out. Supplies and equipment, paper and everything. It was no comparison. [In the Philippines], it was so limited all the time."[78]

The EVP produced many unexpected outcomes. In some cases, returning exchange nurses fulfilled American nurses' expectations by publicizing the achievements of American nursing in the Philippines. However,
their belief in the superiority of American nursing also led to the development of a prejudice among Filipino exchange nurses against Philippine nursing. In 1963, Sofronia Sanchez wrote to the editor of the *PJN,*
"I am a recent arrival from abroad and am now teaching in a school of
nursing. One subject I am interested in is Professional Adjustments. In
my readings around, I have yet to see a local textbook on the subject. . . .
Is this *how backward we are?*"[79]

These attitudes contributed to returnees' desire to go back to the
United States and to some exchange nurses' refusal to leave the United
States at all. In 1963, the FNA observed, "[The Exchange Visitor Pro-
gram] is intended, moreover, to make use of such benefits to our local
areas, upon the return of the nurses privileged to go abroad. What does
happen, however, is the reverse. They seldom desire to come home and
serve our people and our country. They would do anything to prolong
their stay, if not to stay there forever."[80]

Philippine government officials and nursing leaders responded to
these unexpected outcomes of the program in mixed and seemingly contradictory ways. They took pride in the professional achievements of
Filipino nurses abroad, and empathized with the nurses' desire to go to
the United States. They also continued to endorse participation in the
EVP, believing that Filipino nurses' training abroad was necessary for
Philippine development into a modern nation. In this way, Philippine
government officials and nursing leaders seemingly echoed again U.S.
colonial narratives about Filipino backwardness and the modernizing
powers of Western medicine. However, although such a rhetorical move
suggests self-deprecation, Philippine nursing leaders interpreted Filipino
backwardness as a lower-class and rural, as opposed to racial, problem.
Thus, this interpretative shift also echoed the ways American colonial
narratives about health had been refashioned by Western-educated Filipino physicians in the early twentieth century to emphasize class over
racial differences.[81] For example, in 1963, the FNA continued to endorse
participation in the EVP, arguing that "the rural areas, and the towns in
the province are devoid of health leaders who will be willing to dispense
the light of science and of culture over the dark regions of ignorance and

poverty. Only our enterprising young nurses equipped with modern training from abroad, can cope with this need."[82]

At the same time, Philippine government officials and nursing leaders also harshly criticized the new lifestyles of some Filipino exchange nurses abroad. Based on observations in the United States, which claimed that some nurses were "enslaving themselves to the American dollar," government officials and nursing leaders simplified the complexity of Filipino exchange nurses' desires by reducing them to monetary greed.[83] For example, founder and first Dean of the University of the Philippines College of Nursing Julita Sotejo claimed that "money seems to be the sole objective of many exchange visitors. . . . The desire to own a stereo, a huge refrigerator, a modern electric range, and TV set and other electrical appliances has obsessed many a nurse."[84] Critics charged that, as a result of such dangerous obsessions, some Filipino exchange nurses had become financially as well as morally bankrupt. Converting their dollar stipends into pesos, they miscalculated their expenditures that were in U.S. dollars; using credit and layaway plans, they overspent their earnings. In his commencement speech, Paulino Garcia connected these materialist desires with immorality. According to Garcia, money had become an object of worship and had corrupted the nursing profession as well as the nurses themselves: "Will you turn back on your own people when *the almighty dollar* beckons? You must have heard the bitter remarks made by some sectors regarding the reported refusal of most of our nurses who are training abroad, under the Exchange Visitor Program, to come home to serve their people. The chief reason given by such refusal to return home is the incomparably bigger salary such nurses draw in the States. If true, this is indicative of the materialist motive that now *adulterates* the beauty of your profession."[85]

Critics associated the lifestyles of some Filipino exchange nurses in America with licentiousness. They claimed that Filipino exchange nurses smoked, drank, and talked behind each other's back. Julita Sotejo reported, "Cutting each other's throat is a favorite past-time among our kind who work under one roof."[86] The use of marriage to an American citizen to remain in the United States garnered the harshest criticism. In Pura Castrence's commencement speech, she claimed that Filipino exchange nurses abroad "sometimes demeaned themselves by marrying any Tom, Dick or Harry in America, provided Tom, Dick or Harry is an American citizen whose marriage to them would reassure their stay abroad."[87] The editor of the *PJN* likened these nurses, who "marr[ied] any American they could entice, if only to stay in the country of their husbands," to prostitutes: "This is 'selling' themselves."[88]

Filipino exchange nurses participated in these discourses in different ways. Some agreed with these critics; others defended nurses' actions abroad by importantly acknowledging the ways in which U.S. institutional exploitation and discrimination informed these nurses' dollar-earning agendas. As one Filipino exchange nurse argued, "I believe this [exchange] program was designed more to ease the nursing shortage in the United States. The training programs in some hospitals are so inadequate. . . . To compensate for the money and time spent . . . the Filipino nurse . . . tries to earn more money to bring home; hence the unsavory remarks about the Filipino nurse 'enslaving herself to the dollar.' . . . This is not true in all cases, because there were disappointed nurses who asked to be trained in ICUs [intensive care units] and research wards but were not afforded the opportunity."[89]

Just as Philippine government officials and nursing leaders used a rhetoric of spirituality and morality to criticize Filipino exchange nurses, so too did other Filipino nurses, but to reach a very different conclusion. In her speech at a FNA celebration, recent nurse graduate Maribel Carceller connected spiritual sustenance with economic stability and defended work abroad as a spiritual and moral endeavor for herself, her family, and the Philippine nation:

> Ladies and Gentleman, I am a nurse. I come from Barrio Concepcion. . . . My townfolks are farmers. . . . I want to serve my people. . . . But what is in store for me here? What will assure me that I will not be abandoned? Will I be able to help an aging mother? How about my brothers and sisters? . . . Will I be able to live as decently as my profession demands? This is half the trouble. Am I accepted in society as other professionals are? . . .
>
> Ladies and Gentlemen. My wants and needs are human. I want to be socially secure. . . . I must live a life worthy of my profession. Will my salary allow this? I do not exchange service for money. But to keep body and soul fit to further the kingdom of God on this earth, I must be secure. That is why I take the first opportunity to go abroad. . . .
>
> Have I forgotten the ideal of nursing? . . . Have I turned my back on

trembling hands stretched out for help? Have I given [up] hope that my country could prosper with my help? No. But to improve our nation, we must first discipline and improve ourselves. I leave to broaden my outlook, aid my family financially, advance in my nursing experience and come back to the obscure toil and grind of a nurse, earning one-fourth of what I luxuriously enjoyed but for a brief moment.[90]

Philippine government officials, nursing leaders, exchange nurses, and nurse graduates interpreted the exchange visitor experience in multiple and contradictory ways. Their critiques of the EVP coexisted with their continued participation in and endorsement of the program. In these discourses, Philippine as well as American nurses, hospital administrators, and government officials were targets of harsh criticism. Yet all of these groups continued to support the phenomena which brought them together in the first place: the internationalization of nursing and the worldwide mobility of Filipino nurses.

Although the ANA had publicized its concern about EVP abuses in a 1960 statement, the organization continued to promote opportunities for foreign nurses to visit the United States. In 1962, it distributed a brochure to professional nursing organizations worldwide, appropriately entitled "Your Cap Is a Passport." Featuring the faces of women wearing nursing caps and encircling both sides of the globe, the brochure cover illustrated the theoretical underpinnings of, as well as the physical mobility associated with, international nurse migration.[91] Theoretically, the nursing cap (the symbol of professional nursing) enabled these women to practice nursing anywhere in the world. By the 1960s, professional nurses from around the world traveled across national borders under the auspices of various international programs. The 1962 ANA brochure outlined several means through which foreign nurses were able to visit the United States. Aside from the EVP (which the ANA continued to actively participate in, despite its previous statement about the program's abuses), foreign nurses were able to visit the United States through observation programs and full-time academic programs.[92]

For Filipino nurses, their nursing cap was a passport to many parts of the world: Europe, other parts of Asia, the Middle East, North America. In the 1960s, hospitals in Holland, Germany, the Netherlands, Brunei, Laos, Turkey, and Iran also recruited Filipino nurses to alleviate their nursing shortages.[93] Although Filipino nurses had to adjust to different

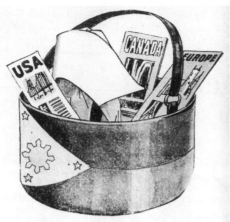

Manila Educational and Exchange Placement Service advertisement in a 1965 issue of the *Philippine Journal of Nursing* portrays travel as a simple route to finding happiness.

languages, kinds of food, and some new nursing procedures, Filipino nursing leaders observed that practices in Europe were in general similar to those in the Philippines.

In the mid-1960s, officers of the FNA visited hospitals in Holland and the Netherlands that had recruited Filipino nurses. Because their reports highlighted the favorable working conditions of nurses working abroad, they functioned, in effect, as recruitment advertisements for nursing overseas. For example, Genara S. M. De Guzman, director of the FNA's International Program, summarized her observations of Filipino nurses working in Holland hospitals this way: "They have good accommodations, classrooms, and facilities. . . . Even student nurses are given individual rooms. Free medical treatment is provided. When nurses get sick they receive 100% full salary even for one year and 80% the second and third year. . . . Nurses work 45 hours a week but this is spread in five days so that they have two regular off days aside from public holidays and vacations. The reception and attention I received from the people I met in Holland are beyond my expectations. . . . The conditions I saw and the atmosphere I felt makes me recommend most unhesitatingly the invitation to our nurses to work in that country."[94]

Similarly, the FNA president reported enthusiastically on the cosmopolitan lifestyle of Filipino nurses and doctors working in Germany: "The Filipino doctors and nurses are provided with a new lovely 5-storey single room apartment each furnished with modern conveniences, kitchenette, bath and toilet. . . . They may cook their food in their own apartments or pay for their lunch in a modern luxurious canteen that serves food Filipinos like. Our Filipino nurses are enjoying their work now as they are given responsible assignments. . . . They are satisfied with their privileges because in addition to the German holidays, they are off on Philippine Holidays, and after 2-week night duty, they are given a week paid holiday which they enjoy traveling to other European cities like Rome, Venice, etc."[95]

In addition to publicizing these favorable work conditions abroad, the FNA continued to associate participation in these international work programs with prestige. The editor of the *PJN* referred to the first group of Filipino nurses in Holland as "the trail-blazers among our colleagues." She endorsed and encouraged this migration overseas by concluding, "The increasing demands for more and more nurses to the Holland area is most satisfying. . . . Let us explore more possibilities and prepare our candidates for this call to world-wide consumership in nursing."[96]

In the mid-1960s, travel advertisements also continued to entice Filipino nurses with opportunities for international sightseeing and employment in the United States and other countries. In one advertisement, Manila Educational & Exchange Placement Service featured a basket decorated with the Philippine flag and adorned with a nursing cap surrounded by travel brochures for the United States, Canada, and Europe. The caption beckoned, "Dear Nurse: . . . Now we have placed over 8,000 nurses to different parts of the world. . . . So, if you're not happy wherever you are right now, why not take the easy way out and go some place else. We can't promise you'll find happiness, but we can help you chase it all over the place. . . . We'll do the worrying and you do the travelling and earning too."[97]

Exploitive hospital employers commodified Filipino nurses as units of labor, but Philippine placement agencies refashioned Filipino nurses' work abroad into a very different kind of commodity. The above advertisement's narrative illustrates the ways in which these agencies represented work abroad as travel, a simple route to fun, adventure, and personal contentment. Although the concept of travel abroad traditionally assumes a definitive period of time outside of one's home country, Filipino exchange nurses also reshaped their work abroad into a very different kind of travel, an indefinite kind of travel that signified socioeconomic success in the Philippines and, as a result of that success, self-redefinition in both the Philippines and the United States. This complex notion of success shaped by Spanish and U.S. colonialism in the Philippines and tempered, though not eliminated, by U.S. exploitation and discrimination would lay the foundation for the increasing migrations and immigration of Filipino nurses in the post-1965 period.

In the 1950s and 1960s, Filipinos and Americans, at times inadvertently and at other times intentionally, transformed a program that was supposed to have been a vehicle for cultural and professional exchange. Unlike the early twentieth-century scholarship programs, the Exchange Visitor Program did not function as a path for occupational mobility in the Philippines. It had become a means to an end. And that end was across the Pacific Ocean. The theme "We shall travel on" in the Filipino Nurses' Hymn began to signify leaving the Philippines for good. In 1965, new U.S. immigration legislation would expedite a phenomenon that was already well underway.

CHAPTER 4

To the Point of No Return

From Exchange Visitor to Permanent Resident

After graduating from Quezon Memorial Hospital School of Nursing, Rosita Macrohon worked at a community clinic in her home province for four years before she came to the United States in 1968. When asked why she left the Philippines, Rosie (as she preferred to be called) responded, "To widen my horizons, to see winter, to see the snow. In the Philippines they say, 'Oh, America is great.'" Initially, Macrohon considered coming to the United States as an exchange nurse, but then changed her mind. She explained, "I went to a travel agency and they told me that instead of coming here on exchange, why don't you come here as a permanent resident? When they told me it's easier to come here as a permanent resident, I waited." After waiting for approximately six months, she received an occupational immigrant visa for the United States.

According to Macrohon, she went to New York City because some of her friends from the Philippines had already settled there, including a nursing school classmate who was an exchange nurse. She applied for work at Columbus Hospital, now called Cabrini Medical Center, because it was located across the street from where some of her friends lived. Within one month of her arrival, Columbus Hospital hired her. "It was very easy," she said.[1]

Macrohon's story reveals that by the late 1960s, Filipino nurses entered the United States through two major avenues: the Exchange Visitor Program and the 1965 Immigration Act's new occupational preferences. The latter avenue enabled Filipino nurses to not only enter the United States but to settle there as permanent residents. Multiple factors contributed to this change. In the United States, the increased demand for nursing services combined with new U.S. immigration policies, including an amendment to the foreign residence requirement of the EVP, facilitated the mass *immigration* of Filipino nurses to the United States.

Macrohon's story also reveals that Filipino nurses applied for new occupational immigrant visas to fulfill desires for travel and adventure in the "great" country of America, and not solely for higher earnings, although this economic incentive would certainly play an important role in Filipino nurse immigration. Although the *individual* stories of Filipino nurse immigrants illustrate an important diversity among this group, this chapter emphasizes that the desires of post-1965 Filipino nurse immigrants like Macrohon were also *collective* desires. Together, Filipino nurse immigrants, whether as nursing school classmates, colleagues, or friends, imagined what America would be like, shared news about recruiting agencies and immigration opportunities, filled out immigration applications, traveled to the United States, and settled near one another upon their arrival there. Macrohon's reference to the presence of one of her nursing school classmates in New York City illustrates one of the ways Filipino nurse immigrants used their own professional networks of support, in particular, networks of Filipino nursing school friends and nurse coworkers, in addition to the more traditional family networks analyzed in migration studies.

The role of the mass media, both print and electronic forms, played an important role in shaping these collective desires. In particular, this chapter analyzes the images and narratives popularized by recruitment advertisements published primarily in the *Philippine Journal of Nursing*. In my emphasis on the collective desires of post-1965 Filipino nurse immigrants and the ways the mass media reflected as well as informed these desires, I resist stereotyping these immigrants' experiences as part of a passive culture that is easily duped by the media to believe in the promise of America. Rather, as Arjun Appadurai points out, "There is growing evidence that the consumption of the mass media throughout the world often provokes resistance, irony, selectivity, and, in general, *agency*. . . . the imagination, especially when collective, can become the fuel for action. It is the imagination, in its collective forms, that creates ideas of . . . higher wages and foreign labor prospects."[2] Furthermore, Filipino nurses' collective desires of "widening one's horizons" by seeing and experiencing "snow and winter," experiences available only outside the national borders of the Philippines, suggest a transnational dynamic of constant change, a dynamic that challenges the concept of culture as an immutable and bounded national, ethnic, and racialized sense of being and belonging.

This chapter expounds on the post-1965 themes touched on in Rosie

Macrohon's narrative: the transition of Filipino nurse migrants' status from exchange nurses to U.S. permanent residents; the continuing significance of social, cultural, and economic motivations for nurses to leave the Philippines to work and live in the United States; the importance of Filipino nurse professional networks in motivating as well as facilitating relocation, employment, and settlement abroad; and the role of Philippine travel agencies as well as U.S. recruitment agencies in the institutionalization of this form of migration. As Jon Goss and Bruce Lindquist have observed, "Labor-scarce economies do not merely create the opportunity for overseas labor to which individual workers respond. . . . The employer and the complex networks of recruitment agencies that link it with the migrant are remarkable in their absence in most accounts of international labor migration."[3] Thus, in the case of post-1965 Filipino nurse immigration, this chapter acknowledges that, whereas the increased demand for nursing services in the United States helped to facilitate this form of mass immigration, an analysis of U.S. hospital employers' and Philippine travel agencies' active recruitment of Filipino nurses as well as the Philippine government's institutionalization of labor export by the mid-1970s provides the necessary international, transnational, and national contexts for understanding the complexity of this mass immigration.

Like the changes that accompanied Filipino nurse migration through the U.S. Exchange Visitor Program, the exodus of Filipino nurses as U.S. immigrants generated controversy in the Philippines as well as the United States. The increasing migration of Filipino nurses abroad continued to be a cause for alarm for nurses and other health personnel in the Philippines. When sentimental appeals to the humanitarianism and the patriotism of Filipino nurses failed, legislative attempts were made to mandate nursing service in Philippine rural areas and to keep new nursing graduates from immediately leaving for work abroad. However, these attempts functioned only as temporary solutions to the major problems of increasingly rapid turnover of nurses in Philippine hospitals and nursing faculty in Philippine schools of nursing.

Furthermore, the interests of Filipino health personnel and the Marcos government diverged. In the early 1970s, the Marcos government began to actively promote the export of Filipino nurses and other Filipino laborers abroad. This new commitment to an export-oriented economy transformed the relationship between nursing and nation building in the Philippines. Filipino nurses working abroad would become the new national heroes through their remittance of desperately needed foreign currency to the Philippines.

TO THE POINT OF NO RETURN

Although the EVP continued to operate through the 1960s, the U.S. government employed other strategies to maintain its image as leader of the "Free World" and to improve its scientific and technological competitiveness with communist countries, specifically the Soviet Union. In 1965, the U.S. Congress passed the Immigration and Nationality Act, which created a more equitable system of immigration. In addition, a major impact of the new legislation was the increased migration of highly educated and skilled persons into the United States.

The Immigration Act of 1965 abolished the national origins system of immigration that had favored the immigration of northern Europeans to the United States, and established a ceiling system involving numerical caps for immigrants from the Eastern and Western Hemispheres.[4] Sending countries in the Eastern Hemisphere were subject to a per country quota of 20,000 immigrants.[5] A preference system determined the distribution of immigrant visas, although immediate family members of U.S. citizens, such as parents, spouses, and minor children, were exempt from these numerical caps.

In the early debates about the structure of the preference system, the Kennedy administration favored the immigration of skilled and educated persons over family members of U.S. citizens. However, the lobbying of organized labor reversed these priorities. The new system included seven preference categories.[6] Reflecting organized labor's preference for family reunification visas over occupational ones, the first, second, fourth, and fifth preference categories were reserved for family members of U.S. citizens and permanent residents. Only two of the seven categories, the third and sixth, applied to skilled immigrants. The third preference category applied to "members of the professions and scientists and artists of exceptional ability"; the sixth applied to "skilled and unskilled workers in occupations for which labor is in short supply." The 1965 Act allotted a maximum of 10 percent of the available visas for each of these categories.

Although the occupational preference categories facilitated the immigration of professionals from all over the world to the United States, Filipino professional immigration in particular played an important role in this migration flow. Between 1966 and 1970, 17,134 Filipino professionals immigrated to the United States, constituting almost one-third of all Filipino immigrants.[7] This contrasted sharply with the average percentage of worldwide professional immigration to the United States. In 1970, for example, professionals from all countries constituted only approximately 11 percent of total immigration to the United States.[8]

Filipino engineers, scientists, and physicians as well as nurses made up the bulk of professional immigrants from the Philippines. From 1966 to 1970, more than 4,300 Filipino engineers and scientists immigrated to the United States.[9] A comparable number of Filipino physicians and nurses immigrated during this five-year period. According to INS statistics, 3,222 Filipino nurses and 2,813 physicians immigrated between 1966 and 1970.[10] However, the total numbers of Filipino heath professionals in the United States during this period were higher than these statistics indicate because Filipino nurses and physicians also entered the United States through other ways, such as the EVP.[11] Between 1966 and 1970, 3,222 Filipino nurses and 2,040 physicians entered the United States with exchange visas.[12]

Although both Filipino physicians and nurses migrated to the United States in significant numbers, nursing emerged as the international specialty of the Philippines. By 1967, the Philippines became the world's top sending country of nurses to the United States, ending decades of numerical domination by European and North American countries. In 1967, Filipino nurses received the highest number of U.S. nursing licenses among foreign-trained nurses, followed by Canadian and then British nurses.[13]

New U.S. legislation also facilitated the adjustment of exchange visitors' status to that of permanent resident. Although separate policies guided the distribution and terms of exchange visitor and immigrant visas, they intersected with the passage of a U.S. public law in 1970. The law provided new grounds that enabled exchange visitors to waive their two-year foreign residency requirement. According to the law, the foreign residency requirement would be applicable in only two situations: first, if the exchange visitor participated in a program financed by the United States or his or her own government; second, if the U.S. Secretary of State designated the exchange visitor's country of origin as clearly requiring the services of the exchange visitor at the time the visitor acquired his or her exchange status.

Congressional hearings revealed that the desires of exchange visitors combined with U.S. demands for exchange visitor labor shaped these amendments to the EVP. According to Congressman Rodino, "The years of experience with the requirement that an exchange visitor must reside in his country of last residence or nationality or a third country for at least two years has, in many instances, resulted in hardship to the exchange visitor." Rodino's comments further reveal that the labor demands of U.S. hospitals informed the new legislation. He continued that "institutions, *particularly hospitals*, have utilized the exchange program more as a vehicle of recruitment than as a basis for training. Evidence before the [Judiciary] committee clearly establishes that many institutions exist primarily with exchange visitor personnel."[14]

Between 1966 and 1978, 7,495 Filipino exchange visitors adjusted their status to become U.S. permanent residents.[15] Milagros Rabara was one of these exchange nurses who was able to adjust her visa status as a result of the new legislation. Rabara arrived in the United States in November 1969 as an exchange nurse at a Chicago hospital. Although she expected her program to last only two years, the amendments took effect while she was in the United States. "Then here comes Nixon," she explained. "He signed a law that . . . we could stay. So that was the good part. So I didn't have to go home."[16]

Rabara applied for permanent residency during the second year of her exchange program. Her characterization of remaining in the United States and no longer returning to the Philippines as "the good part" was one shared by other Filipino exchange nurses. It was also a characterization vigorously promoted by new advertisements in Philippine newspapers and journals recruiting Filipino nurses to work abroad as immigrants as well as exchange visitors.

IMMIGRATION AS TRAVEL AND ADVENTURE

In the late 1960s and early 1970s, Philippine travel agencies and American hospitals continued to actively recruit Filipino nurses for employment in the United States. Their advertisements targeting Filipino nurses reflected the changes in U.S. immigration policy. In 1969, under the caption "Urgent Message to Nurses & Doctors," the House of Travel Incorporated advertised immediate hospital placements in the United States and Canada for "exchange visitors and immigrants." In a 1970 advertisement, the North American Placement & Visa Services, Inc. requested potential exchange visitor nurses to fill out an "expression of interest coupon." Although the advertisement began with the heading, "Exchange Nurses U.S.A.," it continued, "This coupon may also be used by those nurses desiring permanent employment and who intend to go abroad on an IMMIGRANT VISA."[17]

Other travel agencies targeted returned Filipino exchange nurses who were now potential immigrants, a move that vividly illustrated the significance of the transnational community of Filipino nurses created by the EVP. In 1967, Elising G. Roxas, an overseas placement coordinator, travel agent, and registered nurse, advertised her travel and placement services in two issues of the *PJN* with the heading, "Dear Fellow Nurses." In her advertisements Roxas included a photograph of a group of Filipino nurses and other health personnel carrying a "Bon Voyage, Roxas Medical Group" banner while standing in front of an airplane. These advertisements beckoned Filipino nurses to "Come And Join — Enjoy our low cost group travel, the fellowship and camaraderie of your fellow nurses — make your trip a memorable one — seeing Hong Kong and Tokyo." Aside from offering reasonable airfare and monthly departures, Roxas also highlighted her ability to "expedite travel of former exchange nurses for immigrant visas."[18]

By the late 1960s, individual U.S. hospitals also actively recruited their former exchange nurses who had returned to the Philippines to come back for permanent employment. An advertisement from a Chicago hospital featured the faces of Filipino nurses surrounding the caption: "There's A Job Waiting for You at Michael Reese Hospital, Chicago, Illinois, U.S.A." The advertisement targeted Filipino nurses who were former exchange visitors at Michael Reese Hospital and publicized bonuses such as "interest-free loans for travel expenses, continuous inservice education program, and tuition assistance at any recognized university."[19]

After 1965, many other U.S. hospitals placed advertisements in the *PJN* in their effort to recruit Filipino nurses for permanent employment, including Middlesex General Hospital in New Jersey, Sunny Acres Hospital in Ohio, Cook County Hospital in Illinois, and St. Barnabus Hospital in New York. Other U.S. hospitals worked closely with Philippine

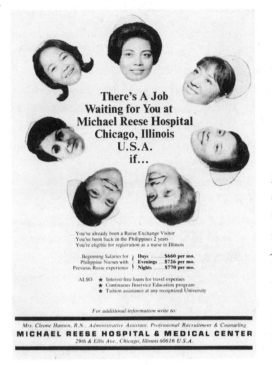

There's A Job
Waiting for You at
Michael Reese Hospital
Chicago, Illinois
U.S.A.
if...

You've already been a Reese Exchange Visitor
You've been back in the Philippines 2 years
You're eligible for registration as a nurse in Illinois

Beginning Salaries for | Days .... $660 per mo.
Philippine Nurses with | Evenings ... $726 per mo.
Previous Reese experience | Nights ..... $770 per mo.

ALSO   ★ Interest-free loans for travel expenses
       ★ Continuous Inservice Education program
       ★ Tuition assistance at any recognized University

For additional information write to:

Mrs. Cleone Hansen, R.N., Administrative Assistant, Professional Recruitment & Counseling
MICHAEL REESE HOSPITAL & MEDICAL CENTER
29th & Ellis Ave., Chicago, Illinois 60616 U.S.A.

Michael Reese Hospital and Medical Center advertisement in a 1969 issue of the *Philippine Journal of Nursing* targets its former exchange visitor nurses from the Philippines for permanent employment.

travel and recruitment agencies. For example, the Philippine placement agency North American Placement and Visa Services, Inc. advertised the visit of American nurse Maureen T. Dreher "representing Beth Israel Hospital in their efforts to recruit immigrant nurses for employment in the United States."[20]

Although U.S. hospitals did not offer Filipino immigrant nurses sight-seeing stopovers in Hong Kong and Tokyo, they did utilize a rhetoric that represented work abroad as travel and adventure in order to attract Filipino nurses. In their advertisements, U.S. recruiters highlighted the hospital's geographic location in the United States, portraying it as exciting, prestigious, and ideal for further travel. For example, in the center of a 1967 Cook County Hospital advertisement was an outline of a map of the United States with a star indicating Chicago. Lines projected out from the star to indicate the location of major cities: New York City, Miami, Dallas, Mexico City, San Francisco, Portland, Seattle, and Toronto. This drawing visually illustrated Cook County Hospital's claim in its advertisement that it was "located in the heart of Chicago —

the nation's transportation hub." Similarly, New York City Health & Hospitals Corporation's advertisement emphasized the thrill of working in New York City. Featuring the Brooklyn Bridge and Manhattan skyline of skyscrapers, the recruitment division of the corporation claimed, "We will help you cross the BRIDGE from where you are to where you want to be . . . NEW YORK CITY! No matter where you are—your nursing diploma can bring you to New York City . . . Imagine! Living and working in America's most exciting city . . . where the whole world looks for the finest medical care!"[21]

The personal narratives of Filipino nurses who immigrated during this time echo the sentiments expressed in these advertisements. After graduating with a Bachelor of Science in Nursing from Far Eastern University in 1968, Elizabeth Kobeckis worked at a city hospital for only one year before applying for an immigrant visa together with nurse-friends who had completed the EVP. She related, "It's not that I was not happy. It's nice working there [in the Philippines]. But of course I wanted to be adventurous and I always want to travel. So I had some friends in the hospital . . . I went with [them] when we applied . . . nurses who had been here before on the exchange visitor [program]. Then they went back there [to the Philippines]. Then they worked. Then they applied for an immigrant visa."[22]

The excitement and energy of Filipino nurses who were applying for immigrant visas inspired their colleagues and friends to apply. Phoebe Cabotaje-Andes immigrated to the United States in 1967. At the time of her visa application, Cabotaje-Andes taught at the Far Eastern University Institute of Nursing. She described her visa application experience animatedly: "One of the faculty of FEU went to the American embassy because she's never been here in the United States. One day she came back with five applications or ten applications, and she said, 'Oh, who wants to go to the United States?'" As Cabotaje-Andes reenacted the part of the faculty member, her voice filled with urgency and she waved her arm in the air as though she were displaying the ten visa applications in her hand. She continued, "She was giving the applications like that. And then we were writing. We were all writing up. 'When are you going back to the embassy?' [we asked]. 'I am going back next week,' [she said]. So we filled [the applications] up. 'Okay, give this,' [we said]. So we hand-carried [the applications back to the embassy] and then in three months we all got accepted."[23]

After passing her nursing board examination in 1966, Corazon Guillermo worked as a staff nurse at Philippine General Hospital before she became hospitalized with a rheumatic heart. Cora (as she preferred to be called) reminisced, "Most of my roommates were leaving the Philippines. . . . In fact I escaped [from the hospital] three times going to the airport to see my friends off." She related that after most of her roommates returned to the Philippines after participating in the EVP, her best friend suggested that they apply together for visas to go abroad. Although her friend completed her visa application, Guillermo did not pursue the matter further because of medical concerns. Later, another friend who was also working at Philippine General Hospital encouraged her to apply: " 'Cora, why don't you come with us? We can apply, just try!' I said, 'No, I might not pass the medical exam. . . . I just don't want to be disappointed, so why should I apply?' [My friend responded,] 'Anyway, why don't you come to the travel agency? Let's go!' " Guillermo eventually immigrated to the United States in 1970. She claimed, "In fact, I was not really sure of my coming here. My family said, 'Why should you go? You don't know how to cook. You don't know how to do this, how to do that. You'll be doing everything.' " However, returning nurses from the EVP largely informed her decision to go to the United States. She explained, "But you know what really happened with me [was that] I envied them for coming here. I really wanted to see the States. That was one of my goals. . . . And when they were coming back, I said, you know, I'm the only one who's not going abroad. And they keep asking, 'Cora, aren't you going here and there? Go there, you have an experience, then you can travel, and all these things.' So you know, with everything that they were telling me, I said I might as well go."[24]

Filipino nursing students also applied for immigrant visas in groups. When Mutya Gener applied for her visa in the mid-1960s, she was still a nursing student at the University of the Philippines College of Nursing. Gener claimed, "I didn't want to come to the U.S. It never entered my mind. . . . My classmates and I . . . there were four of us, friends. . . . So they said, 'Mutya, come on, let's go to America.' It was the fad. . . . So I went. I just wanted the experience of going with them."[25]

According to Rosario-May Mayor, the "fad" of going to the United States continued among Filipino nursing students through the early 1970s. May (as she preferred to be called) arrived in the United States in 1971. She explained, "I got carried on the wave of the gang, like a cohort of friends wanting to come to the United States for adventure, fun, no real objective to make money or that kind of thing. It was just an adventure. The United States was something that everybody was doing. It looks like it's exciting, fun, adventure, more along those lines, not economic. . . . Yes, it's a wave. Let's go to that agency! Let's see this! It's a wave, like twenty of us. We go to parties and all you hear is, 'Oh, there's this recruiting agency!' "26

Mayor's story reveals that the fad of going abroad to the United States attracted even those Filipino nursing students with affluent socioeconomic backgrounds in the Philippines. Mayor was one of those who had experienced a privileged upbringing in the Philippines. She had studied at the exclusive Sta. Scholastica's school system from kindergarten through high school. Both of her parents were health professionals, her father a doctor, and her mother a nurse. Mayor described them as "power brokers in the community." Nevertheless, she was attracted to a decadent, romanticized image of America, which had been popularized by mass media. She reminisced, "This is America and I thought it was going to be all roses and that kind of thing. . . . I think it's the influence of movies that you see, like *Gidget*, Elvis Presley movies, *Casablanca* and Scarlett O'Hara, all that wonderful, you know, Hershey's and M&Ms, all those associations of the good life in America."27

American movies also played a role in Cora Guillermo's decision to go abroad to the United States. When asked why she wanted to go to the United States in particular, she responded, "You see it in the movies. . . . I would like to see Paul Newman. . . . [The United States] must be a great place. I never thought they would have people on the street, homeless people. I never thought that. I thought everything was grand here, that everybody was living well."28

NO BRAIN DRAIN, JUST NO JOB OPPORTUNITY

Although themes of travel and adventure greatly attracted Filipino nurses of various socioeconomic backgrounds to live and work in the United States, their mass immigration was also linked to the persistence of poor working conditions of nurses in the Philippines. Some Philippine newspaper editorials claimed that the mass migration of Filipino nurses abroad through the EVP was "no brain drain."29 Rather, the absence of job opportunities for nurses compelled them to find employment and professional satisfaction outside of the country. Filipino nursing leaders reaffirmed these conclusions. After acknowledging the "growing concern" over the mass exodus of Filipino professionals abroad, Filipino nurse educator Conchita B. Ruiz posed the question, "But is there a so-called brain drain from our shores?" Ruiz urged her readers to consider the unemployment "in the thousands" in the Philippines, the low wages of Filipino government employees, and their poor working conditions in "inadequate facilities." She concluded that "for the present it is evident that in reality, there is no 'brain drain' from the Philippines."[30]

A 1972 survey of 147 Filipino nurses working in Illinois, Minnesota, Montreal, New York, Ohio, and Pennsylvania revealed their dissatisfactions with nursing in the Philippines. When asked if their salaries in the Philippines were commensurate with their professional status and responsibilities, the vast majority, 101 of 147 nurses, responded no; 103 nurses claimed that they did not receive compensation for late shift work, and 102 responded that they did not receive compensation for working on holidays. Slightly more than half of the respondents reported that they had not been paid for overtime and that their hospitals had not followed the forty-hour labor law.[31] One question on the survey asked Filipino nurses if they believed that the nursing profession in the Philippines was faltering and then requested them to list the reasons why or why not. The overwhelming number of responses were affirmative. Among the primary reasons listed for the decline of the nursing profession in the Philippines were the *padrino* system, low salary, and poor working conditions and benefits. The padrino system, also referred to as the *compadre* system, involves the influence of Philippine government officials in the employment opportunities of nurses and other health professionals in hospitals and schools of nursing.

Some of the Filipino nurses I interviewed who immigrated to the United States in the late 1960s and early 1970s expressed similar dissatisfactions. Exchange nurse Epi Mercado, whose story introduced the previous chapter, returned to the Philippines in 1969. She explained that the U.S. government compelled her to return to the Philippines because "her country needed her."[32] She departed from the United States voluntarily and, on her return to the Philippines, applied for work at a government hospital. When the hospital informed her that she needed a recommendation from a Philippine Congress member to secure employment, Mercado claimed that she was "a bit pissed off" at this use of the padrino system and consequently applied for an immigrant visa for the United States. She returned as an immigrant in 1971.

Filipino nurse immigrants I interviewed also cited low wages and the lack of professional opportunities in the Philippines among their major motivations for leaving the country. Elizabeth Kobeckis applied for a travel loan to pay for her airfare before immigrating to the United States in 1971. She explained, "I had to take a loan. . . . You can't afford to live on the salary that you're getting there."[33] Flocerfida Evangelista, who arrived in the United States in 1972, echoed those sentiments: "Back home your salary is so little. . . . Back home tellers at the bank make more money than you."[34]

Despite the financial opportunities available in the United States, the relocation abroad was a difficult process for those Filipino nurses who had earned supervisory positions in Philippine hospitals and schools of nursing. Esther Simpson earned her Bachelor of Science in Nursing from St. Paul College in 1967 and then her Master of Arts degree from the University of the Philippines in 1972. Esther worked at Manila Medical Center while studying for her master's degree and eventually became head of her department. She expressed ambivalence about her decision to immigrate to the United States in 1973:

> I wouldn't have left the Philippines in the first place if the opportunities had been much better, like salary, benefits, insurance coverage, and being able to have material things like we have here in the U.S. If the Philippines were as industrialized and as advanced and if their hospitals were more equipped technically, I would have just stayed there. Manila Medical Center was one of the most advanced hospitals in Manila. I was also teaching at St. Paul's College. I was head of the Inservice Department; it was a prestigious position. It would be hard to begin again in the U.S. But the salary that I had in the Philippines was just good for myself. Though my parents did not expect me to give them money, it would have been a good consolation to my Mom and Dad to receive something from my salary. But I couldn't really give that much.[35]

In 1970, Philippine Nurses Association President Col. Winnie W. Luzon responded to the lack of respect and job opportunities that had frustrated Filipino nurses. She insisted, "The first thing we will embark on is to try to help every nurse secure a just reward and fair share in the privileges and rights she is entitled to as a professional."[36] Luzon appealed to Filipino nurses to unify under the auspices of the professional organization. However, given its history of internal divisions, Filipino nurses unsurprisingly did not heed her call. In the 1972 survey of Filipino nurses abroad, over a quarter listed "an ineffective PNA" as one of the reasons for the decline of the nursing profession in the Philippines. And some nurses in the Philippines abandoned their profession altogether to engage in more financially lucrative employment. A 1973 survey of Filipino massage attendants revealed that many were former nurses.[37]

Advertisements for U.S. hospitals took advantage of the economic and professional dissatisfaction of nurses in the Philippines to recruit them to work in their institutions. In its 1967 advertisement, Chicago's Cook County Hospital encouraged Filipino nurses to "Get Up and Go to Cook County Hospital where you can earn from $570 TO $845 A MONTH." The hospital strategically printed the monthly salary range in an extra large font size. The advertisement for Michael Reese Hospital featured the hospital's "beginning salaries for Philippine nurses with previous Reese experience." It claimed that they would earn $660 per month for day shift work, $726 per month for nights, and $770 per month for evenings.[38]

Appealing to Filipino nurses' desire for professional opportunities, recruitment advertisements emphasized hospitals' up-to-date medical facilities and continuing education opportunities. Cook County Hospital boasted that its nurses would work "using the most modern equipment and employing the latest techniques." Middlesex General Hospital's advertisement characterized the hospital as a "modern 280 bed teaching hospital" that offered registered nurses a tuition plan and continuing education programs.[39] The recruitment advertisements of U.S. hospitals also publicized other socioeconomic bonuses that the majority of Filipino nurses working in the Philippines did not enjoy: uniform allowances, health plans, pension plans, weekends off, paid vacations, holidays, and sick leave. Finally, they expressed respect for nurses with captions such as: "Imagine! . . . Putting your professional skills to work where they're appreciated and needed."[40]

FILIPINO NURSE NETWORKS

Filipino nurses immigrated as cohorts. They applied for immigrant visas together. They also arranged their travel itineraries together. For example, when Delia Hernandez (not her real name) learned that two of her classmates from the University of the Philippines College of Nursing were immigrating to the United States at around the same time in 1970, the three of them decided to coordinate their itineraries and fly to the United States together. A classmate's sister, who was a travel agent, arranged their travel plans.[41]

Unlike Filipino exchange nurses, who arrived in the United States under the sponsorship of a specific hospital, immigrant nurses often came to the United States without prearranged employment. As a result, they actively sought the company of nursing friends and family members who could help them with the adjustment process. Delia Hernandez's destination was New York City because her aunt had previously settled there. Hernandez and one of her classmates lived with her aunt before eventually finding work at the same hospital in Manhattan and their own housing. Esther Simpson's first destination was Chicago because her aunt and sister, who were both nurses, resided there.

Although Filipino nurses went elsewhere if they were dissatisfied with their living conditions, they often relocated to other areas in the United States where other nursing friends and relatives had settled. For example, after working as a staff nurse in San Pablo Hospital for many years, Mercedes Alcantara immigrated to the United States in 1972. Her first destination was Michigan, where her brother lived. She was able to find employment, but she disliked living in Michigan. She contacted two nursing friends she had worked with in San Pablo Hospital in the Philippines, who were then residing in New York City. The presence of her two nursing friends in New York City motivated her to relocate there in 1974. The three of them shared an apartment in an area located conveniently near all of their hospital employers.[42]

Filipino nurse networks also extended into the area of employment. When Lolita Compas immigrated to the United States in 1969, her older sister was already working as a nurse at New York City's Cabrini Medical Center. Although her sister had left the nursing profession by the time Compas arrived, according to her, working at Cabrini was "a given."

Former exchange visitor nurses who returned to the United States as immigrants utilized contacts from their exchange visitor experience. As an exchange nurse, Epi Mercado had worked and studied under the auspices of New York University's oncological nursing program, a program affiliated with James Ewing Hospital. When she returned to New York City as an immigrant she found employment at the Memorial Sloan-Kettering Cancer Center, which she described as "a sister hospital of James Ewing Hospital." According to her, she had applied for work at the cancer center while she was an exchange nurse, and on her return to the United States, the hospital still had her records.[43]

The location of the hospital as well as the presence of Filipino nursing friends influenced their job searches and decisions. Esther Simpson described her experience of finding work this way: "The hospital yellow pages in Chicago is about ten pages and so I chose the ones that were close." The hospital she eventually decided on was only five blocks away from where she lived. Simpson added, "And that's where I had some friends from the Philippines and so I went ahead and started there." Lolita Compas claimed that many Filipino nurses and other health workers were attracted to work at Cabrini Medical Center because Filipinos constituted a significant percentage of the hospital staff. According to her, Cabrini Hospital is sometimes referred to as "Manila General" because of their large numbers, and, as a result, Cabrini provides Filipino employees with "a sense of belonging." Compas explained, "People gravitate where there are a lot of your own kind. It's like a second home. You have no relatives, so your friends and your colleagues become your extended family."[44]

The majority of newly arrived Filipino nurse immigrants I interviewed were single at the time of immigration; a few had already been married in the Philippines. They sponsored their husbands to come to the United States with them.[45] Although the husbands' initial reaction to migration abroad varied, the wives claimed that once they had received their immigrant visas, there was little debate about whether they would relocate abroad. According to Phoebe Cabotaje-Andes, immigrant nurses had a deadline by which they had to accept or reject the visa. After the U.S. government approved her visa, she related, "I told my husband, I said, 'You know, I'm going to the States.' 'What?!' [he said]. 'Yeah, I'm going to the States. I am approved,' [I said]. . . . In six months time, we all came. Then my husband followed."[46]

The reactions of Elizabeth Kobeckis's and Mutya Gener's husbands reflect the broad spectrum of responses to Filipino nurse wives' new immigrant status. Kobeckis's husband accompanied her to the United States in 1971, but, according to her, he did so unwillingly. He was a mechanical engineer who was working in a private firm at the time. She related, "He doesn't even want to come with me. But since we are married, he has no choice. So he has to come with me and see what is here, whether we are coming here or we're coming back." She and her husband temporarily resided with his parents in Brooklyn, New York. After they had both found jobs, they decided to live across the street from his parents. Kobeckis explained that she had become pregnant and that her relatives helped take care of their child when she went back to work. "It's like a family arrangement," she said. "It's hard to be here without anybody, without knowing anybody."[47]

By contrast, Mutya Gener claimed that her husband encouraged her to go to the United States; he wanted to be an artist. Gener herself had graduated with a Bachelor of Arts in Music from Silliman University before her mother "coerced" her into studying nursing. In the United States, Gener explained, a person could "reinvent" himself or herself. She described their decision to immigrate abroad together romantically: "My husband had a very good job [in the Philippines]. He was a lawyer. He was a [University of the Philippines] graduate. He was earning a lot but he hated it. A steel corporation, he was the legal consultant. He always wanted to be a writer. He was coerced to be a lawyer. So we met, it was like destiny. He's a very quiet man, reads a lot of books. He said, 'Mutya, since it's easy for us, you can go the States, let's go.' So we did."[48]

In addition to the professional and family networks utilized by Filipino nurse immigrants, U.S. labor demands facilitated Filipino nurse employment and settlement. Many of the nurses I interviewed who immigrated during this time characterized obtaining a U.S. occupational immigrant visa and finding employment in the United States as an "easy" process that took no longer than several months. Phoebe Cabotaje-Andes related, "It was so easy. Just one day, it just opened, third preference." Mutya Gener claimed that in the late 1960s "it was easy to come here on the third preference [visa]. . . . They really needed nurses here."[49] U.S. hospitals needed the services of foreign-trained nurses because the demand for nursing services increased and because domestic nursing shortages continued to leave these services unfulfilled. The establishment of two public health programs, Medicare for the elderly and Medicaid for the poor, in 1965 rapidly increased the demand for health care. Meanwhile, in 1967 the National League for Nursing cited a shortage of 125,000 nurses in the United States.[50] Gener continued, "[American hospitals] needed you. They didn't care whether you're an alien with six eyes as long as you can do nursing."

NEW AVENUES, NEW PROBLEMS

The increasing exodus of Filipino nurses through new avenues of immigration created new problems for nursing in the Philippines. These included the exponential growth of schools of nursing, the rapid turnover of Philippine nursing faculty, and the dissolution of Philippine nursing organizations. As the demand for nursing education exceeded the enrollment spaces available in Philippine colleges and schools of nursing beginning in the early 1960s, Filipino entrepreneurs opened new schools of nursing in the provinces as well as urban areas. Between 1950 and 1970 the number of nursing schools in the Philippines rose from 17 to 140.[51] In 1966 Philippine Republic Act 4704 relaxed the minimum standards for nursing school operation.[52] Previously, the government required a school of nursing to maintain one hundred hospital beds as well as provide an adequate library, classrooms, and teaching equipment and supplies. Under the 1966 Act, the government allowed the establishment of schools of nursing with fifty hospital beds, as long as these schools affiliated with other hospitals to provide for the remaining balance necessary to meet the one hundred–bed minimum.

The increase in nursing schools continued through the mid-1970s because the owners of these schools earned huge profits from the tuition and other related expenses of their students. In the 1972 survey of 147 Filipino nurses working abroad, the overwhelming majority (130) claimed that the total cost of nursing education in the Philippines was too high.[53] Leonor Malay Aragon, dean of the University of the Philippines College of Nursing, lamented:

Despite our Herculean efforts to stop the opening of more and more colleges and schools, we are helpless because the hospitals that open these schools are owned by doctors who as a group are very strong and powerful.

One of the biggest headaches we face in nursing education is the high cost of nursing education. It has become one of the most expensive careers for girls to take and a most profitable one for the hospital owners. Where girls in this country were paid before to take up Nursing and given to all kinds of inducements like free board and lodging, they now pay huge sums — to the hospitals for affiliation fees, books, board and lodging. Indeed, the possibilities of making money through a nursing school is limitless. And the free service that students render to patients while learning is not even given value in the final cost of accounting. Since they spend so much for their education, naturally their tendency after graduation is to go abroad.[54]

As the number of nursing schools increased, so too did the demand for nursing school faculty. Yet, the rapid turnover of Philippine nursing faculty ensued as the socioeconomic rewards of working abroad also attracted nursing instructors. Although the Philippine Board of Examiners for Nurses required a ratio of one faculty member to ten to twelve students during clinical supervision, according to one nursing dean, Rosario S. Diamante, the ratio was "not possible due to the rapid turn-over of faculty. This was mainly due to an exodus abroad either as immigrant or as participant of the Exchange Visitors Program or under a working visa."[55] A 1974 summary of problems encountered by the Council of Deans and Principals of Philippine Colleges and Schools of Nursing, Inc. included the "sprouting of many schools of nursing posing problems of lack of qualified faculty members." According to the Council, "We conduct seminars for them only to find out that they have left the country."[56]

In the late 1960s and early 1970s, although Philippine nursing leaders criticized the mass exodus of Filipino nurses abroad and its devastating effect on the state of Philippine nursing education and service, they themselves were not immune to the attractions of work abroad. Filipino nursing leaders founded the Association of Nursing Service Administrators of the Philippines (ANSAP) in 1968. However, the organization dissolved as "the leaders who spear-headed the organization left one by one for abroad."[57]

In 1973, a Philippine Nurses Association board member organized a workshop attended by chief nurses, nursing service directors, and government and private hospital supervisors to reactivate ANSAP. By the end of the three-day workshop, the participants elected officers for the revived organization and adopted the original constitution and bylaws. Enthusiasm was high as approximately 250 Filipino nursing leaders attended the workshop. On the organization's first anniversary in 1974, approximately 360 Filipino nurses attended ANSAP's one-day symposium. They discussed the same problems that had plagued Filipino nurses and nursing administrators since the late 1960s: "inadequate and ineffective nursing education, lack of nurses, lack of leadership, rapid turnover of nurses, low salary, communication gap between hospital administrators and hospital owners." The association's president, Perla Sanchez, lamented that nursing administrators in the Philippines continued to compete with the active recruitment of Filipino nurses abroad: "We seem to be in a situation in which nursing seems to be directless. We are losing nurses and we are losing nurses faster than we produce them. Those who have left and returned and those who have stayed are becoming discontented and fraught with frustration."[58]

In the 1950s and early 1960s, the mass migration of Filipino nurses through the EVP provoked sentimental pleas from nursing leaders and government officials to nurse graduates to return and to serve the people of the Philippines. As new avenues of entry to the United States only exacerbated the trend of migration abroad, as the aggressive international recruitment of Filipino nurses continued unabated, and as nurse wages in the Philippines lagged pathetically behind those of nurses abroad, Filipino nursing leaders in collaboration with the Philippine government employed new strategies to retain nurse graduates, if only temporarily. In the early 1970s, mandatory health service requirements for new nurse graduates replaced emotional appeals to nurses' selflessness and humanitarianism.

These service requirements were short term. For example, in 1972, the Philippine Exchange Visitor Program Committee required medical and nursing graduates to serve in the Philippines for one year after the results of their board examinations before applying to the exchange program.[59] In 1973, President Ferdinand Marcos issued a presidential decree requiring nurse graduates to work four months in a rural area as a condition for obtaining licensure.[60]

The purpose of these service requirements was to alleviate general nursing shortages in the Philippines, specifically the urban versus rural maldistribution of nurses within the country. Marcos and the PNA presidents justified mandatory health service requirements by comparing the nurse-to-patient ratios in the Philippines with those in other countries. The Philippines' ratio was 8 nurses for every 10,000 people; Canada's was

57 for every 10,000; West Germany, 27 for every 10,000; and the United States, 49 for every 10,000. The irony was not lost on PNA President Fe Valdez, who observed, "These are the countries that are importing our nurses, yet their ratio is more than what we presently have."[61] Of the nurses working in the Philippines, only approximately one-third served in rural areas. This maldistribution resulted in an even more imbalanced nurse-to-patient ratio in rural areas; 1 nurse for every 33,000 people.

According to the service requirement guidelines, Filipino medical and nursing graduates were able to select three places in which to serve. However, a system of drawing lots determined their service area if too many graduates chose the same place. Their service requirement took place during the four-month waiting period for their board results.[62] The Philippine government paid for some expenses and provided a minimal stipend for the service. Nurse graduates received free transportation to the place of assignment, a stipend of 150 pesos per month for board and lodging, and a daily allowance of 5 pesos.

FROM EXCHANGE TO EXPORT OF *WOMAN*POWER

Ferdinand Marcos's decrees mandating several months of health service in rural areas were token gestures to alleviate the maldistribution of health personnel in the country. At the same time Marcos issued these decrees, he also committed the Philippine government and economy to a new model of development based on export-oriented industrialization. His commitment to an export-oriented economy included the export of people as well as goods. Both forms were rife with contradictions. The Marcos government promoted a massive export of agricultural goods while many Filipinos suffered from rural landlessness and malnutrition.[63] Government officials also promoted the export of laborers, including nurses, when the ratios of Filipino nurses serving the general population were abysmal.

Philippine government officials began to take notice of overseas migrant laborers in the late 1960s.[64] Whereas the government of the 1950s and 1960s promoted the "exchange" of Filipino visitors for cultural and technological reasons, by the early 1970s it promoted "employment contracts" of Filipino laborers and a "dollar repatriation program." Through these measures, the Marcos government attempted simultaneously to alleviate unemployment in the Philippines and to revitalize a flailing economy. Although Filipino male laborers, in particular loggers working in Kalimantan, Indonesia and construction workers employed by U.S. military bases in Vietnam and Thailand, initially captured the attention of Philippine government officials, they also observed the overseas demand for women workers, mainly nurses. Marcos's address to the PNA at its 1973 convention in Manila revealed this change toward the government's new commitment to exporting *woman*power:

> To protect the Filipino nurses abroad from discrimination and exploitation, I have approved the recommendation of the Dept. of Labor which prepared at my instance, at my orders, and also the Secretary of Health and the PNA to exclude Filipino nurses from the coverage of the RP-US Exchange Visitor Program. . . . This merely means that when you are sent abroad as a student they pay you less than the regular nurses. That is what is happening. And so they keep asking for exchange students and student nurses. And they utilize them the same way as they utilize all other nurses in the hospitals. In fact they are probably working more than the regular nurses, and to me this is a violation of not only the normal ordinary decencies of human relations but it also violates our understanding. So, we would like an arrangement by which when the nurses go, they go by a working visa, that means that their working visa is based on a contract that will cover the relationship. Whereas now, many of the student nurses and visitors abroad are not covered at all by any agreement or contract and so they are exploited by the employer. And so, in short, what is the policy of nursing? . . . It is our policy to promote the migration of nurses. We can allow the migration of nurses. We will allow them to go out, improve themselves, earn money but under the terms and conditions consistent with the dignity of the Filipino people and the Filipino worker in general and the fabled integrity, competence and compassion of the Filipino nurses in particular.

Such expressions of concern for "the dignity of the Filipino worker in general" and "the fabled integrity, competence and compassion of Filipino nurses in particular" attempted to create a humane image of Marcos's labor export policy. But his address also revealed the commodification of Filipino nurses vis-à-vis their mass production for an international market. Marcos continued, "We intend to take care of [Filipino nurses] but as we encourage this migration, I repeat, we will now encourage the training of all nurses because as I repeat, *this is a market* that we should take advantage of. Instead of stopping the nurses from going abroad *why don't we produce more nurses? If they want one thousand nurses we produce a thousand more.*"[65]

The commodification of the Filipino nurse as a product of domestic mass production and a demand of an international marketplace was further compounded by Marcos's monetary aim of foreign currency accumulation through remittances from workers abroad. Like the revenues earned from agricultural exports, Filipino nurses abroad would build the Philippine national economy by depositing their earnings abroad in Philippine banks. Marcos concluded his address by encouraging Filipino nurses abroad to earn for the country as well as for themselves:

> I ask [Filipino nurses abroad] to participate in the dollar repatriation program. . . . You don't lose your money with the dollar repatriation plan. You merely deposit it with a bank that has a correspondent here and [where] you have a deposit bag. . . . help your country by putting your money in a bank in the Philippines so that your money will earn for you and earn for the country at the same time. When you put your money in a foreign bank, you are helping [the] foreign bank to earn money. Probably they don't need it. . . . But here we need every dollar that we can get our hands on, in order to increase our industrialization program. . . . Because every dollar that you utilize in this manner helps and contributes meaningfully to our economic development by keeping our dollar reserves at their present unprecedented high level.[66]

Given the shift to an export-oriented economy, Filipino nurses abroad no longer abandoned their role in Philippine nation building but became integral to it. Once criticized by the Philippine Secretary of Health in the mid-1960s for "turning their backs on their own people when the almighty dollar beckons," Filipino nurses working abroad and earning dollars became the Philippines' new national heroes.[67] In his 1973 address to visiting Filipino nurses from abroad, a new Philippine Secretary of Health, Clemente S. Gatmaitan, proclaimed:

> As head of the Health Department, I consider you as "Long-Lost Daughters"—prodigal children so to speak, who have returned temporarily to the fold. Personally, I wish you for good. But on second thought, we in the Health Department are happy that you have elected to stay and work abroad. . . . First of all, you project an excellent image of our country and our people. While in other countries, you give prestige to the Philippines

because you are all virtually ambassadors of good will. We receive glowing reports from abroad that Filipina Nurses are preferred to nurses of other nationalities because of inherent sterling qualities that make you ideal members of the Nursing Profession, this is an honor for all of you and this, in turn, honors us here at home. For this, we are proud of you. Another benefit that accrues from your work is the precious dollar you earn and send back to your folks at home. In this manner, you help indirectly in the improvement of our economic condition.[68]

These changes in Philippine government officials' attitudes toward the mass migration of Filipino workers abroad led to the implementation of an official overseas labor policy. In 1974, the government created the Overseas Employment Development Board. This agency publicized the availability of Filipino labor in overseas labor markets, evaluated overseas employment contracts, and recruited Filipino laborers for work abroad.

By the mid-1970s Asian professional immigrants in the United States numerically dominated those from other parts of the world. Between 1970 and 1974, INS statistics reveal that 42,503 professional immigrants came from Asia. The second major sending geographic area was North America, with 5,764 professional immigrants. Within this span of five years, only 1,874 professional immigrants came from Europe. Sociologists and other migration scholars observed that the Philippines played an important role in the numerical significance of Asian professional immigrants. Of the 42,503 professional immigrants from Asia, over 50 percent, 26,690 of them, were from the Philippines.[69]

The large number of Filipino nurses migrating to the United States constituted a significant percentage of Filipino professional immigration. In the Philippines, it seemed as though this trend would not only continue but increase. In 1975, *PJN* editors referred to the low salaries and poor working conditions of Filipino nurses as "the age-old gripe." At the closing ceremonies of the PNA's fifty-third Foundation Anniversary in 1975, Philippine Secretary of Labor Blas Ople sympathized with nurses and other medical personnel leaving the Philippines for employment abroad, characterizing the cause of this mass exodus as the "irrationality of investing so much in one's education and recovering so little in terms of returns."[70]

The persistence of low nursing wages and poor working conditions in the Philippines, the emergence of new problems in the Philippine nursing profession, and the Philippine government's active promotion of the migration of nurses combined with the aggressive recruitment of Filipino nurses to work in the United States as well as nurses' own desires for travel and adventure abroad to reaffirm Milagros Rabara's opinion that working and residing permanently in the United States was "the good part." However, in the 1960s and 1970s, American violence complicated romanticized narratives about life in the United States.

PART III

Still the Golden Door?

Such was the enigma of the little Filipino: responsible, considerate, shy.
But was it a veil hiding evil beneath? — ROBERT WILCOX,
The Mysterious Deaths at Ann Arbor, 1976

[The jury] didn't do the right thing. . . . I don't know about American
justice. — LEONORA PEREZ, talking about her and Filipina Narciso's
conviction of conspiracy and poisoning in the VA Hospital murders,
July 1977, in Jim Graham, "Convicted Nurses Are Critical of Jury"

Nurses in this country are fighting for a new image. . . .
These foreign nurses are not members of our professional organization.
They do nothing to further our professional cause!
— American nurse BONNIE VOWELL, criticizing the funding of a
prescreening examination for foreign nurses, in "Why Shouldn't Foreign
Nurses Pay Their Own Way?" 1978

Foreign nurses, particularly Fillippinas [*sic*], are the "COOLIES OF
THE MEDICAL WORLD." . . . I would like to see all foreign nurses
walk out of the hospitals in this country, and see what happens.
— Filipino nurse NORMA RUSPIAN WATSON, writing
to the U.S. Commission on Civil Rights, 1979

CHAPTER 5

Trial and Error

Crime and Punishment in America's "Wound Culture"

While the significant numbers of Filipino nurses abroad caught the attention of U.S. hospital administrators, nursing leaders, and government officials in the 1960s, violence, and not demographics, publicized the presence of Filipino nurses in America to the general public. Americans came to know of Filipino nurses in the United States through two sensational, well-publicized murder cases: the Speck massacre of 1966 and the VA (Veterans Administration) murders of 1975. Both cases involved mass murders in hospital-related contexts that shocked and horrified Americans and Filipinos. However, one major difference was the way in which each case featured Filipino nurses: as victims and then as perpetrators of crime.

In the summer of 1966, Richard Speck murdered eight student nurses in Chicago, including two Filipino exchange nurses, Merlita Gargullo and Valentina Pasion. The lone survivor of this massacre was another Filipino exchange nurse, Corazon Amurao, who would later identify and testify against Speck as the prosecution's star witness. Almost a decade later, in the summer of 1975, the Federal Bureau of Investigation investigated multiple breathing failures at the VA Hospital in Ann Arbor, Michigan. They charged two Filipino nurses, Filipina Narciso and Leonora Perez, who worked at the hospital, with conspiracy, poisoning, and murder. In July 1977 a jury convicted Narciso and Perez of conspiracy and three counts of poisoning. However, in February 1978, the U.S. Attorney dismissed the case against them after the defense team appealed the verdict. This chapter juxtaposes and explores these two murder cases in the context of the changing patterns of Filipino nurse migration in the post-1965 period, the persistence of a culture of U.S. imperialism in the late twentieth century, and what Mark Seltzer has called America's "wound culture," the American public's fascination with serial killing and bodily violence.[1]

An exploration of these two murder cases is significant for several reasons. First, the extreme and opposing situations of Filipino nurses in these two cases — as victims and as alleged perpetrators — and the subsequent seemingly contradictory images of them in American newspapers and popular nonfiction reflect the dynamic complexities of Filipino nurse representations in American society, complexities steeped in a culture of U.S. imperialism. That the cases took place during a time when the visa status of the majority of Filipino nurses in America changed from that of exchange visitor to permanent resident suggests that Filipino nurse representations in America were linked to changing U.S. political, social, and economic contexts. In the mythology of the U.S. Exchange Visitor Program, Filipino exchange nurses were Philippine ambassadors of goodwill. As products of an American-influenced nursing education in the Philippines who aimed to improve themselves even further with postgraduate training in the United States, Speck victims Gargullo and Pasion were evidence of American benevolence and postcolonial promise. The American public mourned their deaths. However, in the 1970s, Filipino nurses no longer intended to return to the Philippines and became U.S. permanent residents in increasingly high numbers. This shift in Filipino nurses' desires and migration patterns became a multifaceted cause for alarm in the United States. Thus, despite their Americanized professional training and needed skills, Filipino immigrant nurses Narciso and Perez emerged as dark, dangerous, and conspiratorial Filipino natives with the propensity to harm their American patients in the context of this politicized demographic change.

Second, the portrayals of the alleged murderers and their victims in popular nonfiction revealed the uneven ways forms of American popular culture portrayed violence committed by white American male Richard Speck and by Filipino immigrant women Filipina Narciso and Leonora Perez. The volume of publicity devoted to mass murderer Speck — his childhood, his lifestyle, his motivations for such a heinous crime — eventually overshadowed that of his victims and surpassed the attention given to the individual lives of alleged VA murderers Narciso and Perez. A comparative analysis of two popular nonfiction books following the Speck massacre and the VA murders about "the untold story of Richard Speck" and "the most chilling medical horror story of our time" reveals that the individuality of Speck as a human being — though a terribly disturbed one — was a prominent feature in this literature, whereas the inscrutability of Narciso and Perez as mysterious Filipinos was highlighted. This contrast highlights the ways the race, gender, and national origin of American mass murderers and serial killers are salient categories that shape the American public's understanding of and reaction to violence.

Mark Seltzer has argued that the very idea of "the public" has become inextricably linked to spectacles of mass violence and that these spectacles have functioned as a way of imagining and situating our notions of public, social, and collective identity.[2] However, the reactions to the Speck massacre and the VA murders suggest that these spectacles shape and reflect multiple publics that are racialized, gendered, and classed. Aside from the mainstream American public, these multiple publics included, but were not limited to, a transnational Filipino public and an Asian American public. In particular, the Filipino protests against the treatment of Narciso and Perez revealed how fractured and tenuous a Filipino community could be. Politically divided over Ferdinand Marcos's recent declaration of martial law in the Philippines, Filipinos in the United States and the Philippines formed a fragile coalition to raise support for the two nurses.

In exploring these representations and narratives of these two sensational cases, I argue that the significance of Filipino nurse migration is more than a unique chapter in the history of contemporary immigration and labor. The phenomenon also provides a useful lens to view the contradictions of late twentieth-century American cultural history — specifically, the American public's obsession with certain kinds of violence and its erasure of U.S. imperial violence.

THE CRIME OF THE CENTURY

On July 14, 1966, in a middle-class neighborhood in southeast Chicago, in a house rented by the South Chicago Community Hospital as a residence for some of its student nurses, Richard Speck murdered eight student nurses. He bound each woman with strips of bedsheet in a bedroom and proceeded to take them outside of the room one at a time. During one of his absences, Filipino exchange nurse Corazon Amurao, with her wrists and ankles bound, rolled herself under one of the bunks against the wall. Amurao later testified that two of the American student nurses gave muffled cries and that one of the Filipino exchange nurses said, *"Masikit"* or "It hurts" in Tagalog as Speck led them outside the room.[3] At around 5:30 the next morning, Amurao freed herself and went from room to room of the house, where she discovered the bodies of her friends. Speck had strangled and stabbed his victims in their necks, chests, hearts, and eyes. Although conflicting reports emerged about the occurrence of sexual assault, some media reports characterized the massacre as a "murder-sex orgy."[4] The Cook County coroner and four major Chicago dailies referred to it as "the crime of the century."[5]

The Speck massacre was a classic example of what Mark Seltzer has called America's "atrocity exhibitions" that constitute "the contemporary pathological public sphere."[6] As police cars arrived at the scene of the crime, one news report observed that "neighbors grabbed housecoats, slipped pants over their pajamas, and hurried out into the street. Police roped off the area around the victims' residence. The crowd started to form. As the news became more widespread the number of spectators swelled into the hundreds."[7] Another report described how many members of the crowd held transistor radios to their ears and strained for news reports of the murder "the way baseball fans sometimes tune in to the game while sitting at the ballpark."[8] Spectators continued to drive by and gather around the scene of the crime days after it occurred. One neighbor claimed, "I've never seen so many 'ghouls' driving by trying to get a look at the house and even trying to get in. . . . Why would anyone want to see something like that?"[9]

The massacre brought to crisis mainstream America's racialized, sexualized, and classed assumptions about the safety of its "good" neighborhoods and the "good" women who lived there. As one writer for the *Chicago Daily News* agonized, "How could one man kill eight girls in a civilized neighborhood where the sky is still open and every house has a lawn?"[10] And as one family friend of one of the victims lamented, "I just don't understand it. I could understand it better if the girls were bad girls, but they were all good."[11] A *Chicago Tribune* editorial contrasted the Speck massacre with the 1929 St. Valentine's Day executions, which also took place in Chicago, by noting that the seven men gunned down in that mass murder were "no great loss to the community." By contrast, in the Speck massacre, "the fact that these girls were young, that they embarked on constructive careers, and that they were decent and unoffending enhances the horror of the crime." The racialized and classed assumptions about the goodness of Speck's victims appeared later in the editorial, as the author criticized Chicago "street mobs" and a "'civil rights' spokesman" from distracting police with their cries of "police brutality." According to the editorial, such distractions diverted the energies of police who were trying to apprehend the nurses' murderer.[12]

Jeffery Manor, the neighborhood in which the murders took place, boasted the racialized, sexualized, and classed features of idyllic, suburban America: white, heterosexual, middle-class families seeking new homes after World War II "away from the crowded old neighborhoods of Chicago."[13] The neighborhood had a population of approximately 7,500 people who lived primarily in single-family brick bungalows. According to one police sergeant, "Bicycle thefts are a greater problem here than mugging or any kind of violence."[14] It seemed an ideal site for a nursing residence, a place that provided a safe environment for middle-class young women studying and practicing nursing in urban areas.

Six of Speck's victims were white American senior nursing students who were scheduled to graduate in early August. Gloria Davy, Suzanne Farris, Mary Ann Jordan, Patricia Matusek, Nina Schmale, and Pamela Wilkening were in their early twenties. Local residents described them as nice, quiet, and pretty. The U.S. media portrayed them as all-American girls, local heroines committed to serving their communities and the nation. Several of them were from the Midwest and had been volunteers, athletic champions, and teachers in their hometowns. Twenty-two-year-old Davy worked as a nurse's aide at Our Lady of Mercy Hospital in Dyer, Indiana, and later became president of the Illinois Student Nurses Association. She had been the head of the cheerleading squad and a "Sweetheart of the Future Farmers of America" at her high school. Twenty-year-old Matusek had been a local swimming champion and water ballet team member. Twenty-four-year-old Schmale was a former Sunday school teacher in Wheaton, Illinois. Their plans after graduation reflected their commitment to caregiving, civic service, and family. Matusek planned to work at Chicago Children's Memorial Hospital after her training, and Davy intended to join the Peace Corps. In addition to pursuing nursing after graduation, Schmale and Farris were engaged to be married. Jordan did not live in the student nurses' house, but visited that night to help Farris make wedding plans. Farris was engaged to be married to Jordan's brother.

Two of Speck's victims were Filipino exchange nurses who had recently graduated from nursing programs in the Philippines. Twenty-two-year-old Merlita Gargullo and twenty-three-year-old Valentina Pasion were members of the class of 1965 from Arellano University and Manila Central University, respectively. The U.S. media also portrayed Gargullo and Pasion as "good" girls who were pretty, soft-spoken, and hardworking. Pasion was "full of jokes and well liked among the nurses." Gargullo would "blush whenever a boy approached her."[15] Although they had been in the United States only two months before the massacre occurred, Gargullo and Pasion had followed patterns of other Filipino exchange nurses who wrote letters to their friends and relatives in the Philippines about America as a land of promise. Pasion wrote a younger sister saying that she was enjoying her stay in America so much that she wished she could live there forever.[16] Gargullo wrote a close friend and classmate in the Philippines saying that she was very happy. She had visited Wisconsin, and she was planning to send her friend some perfume and silk stockings.[17]

According to Corazon Amurao, she, Gargullo, and Pasion had initially tried to evade Speck by locking themselves in a bedroom closet. Amurao explained that they joined their hands on the doorknob inside holding the door tightly closed for about five minutes. However, one of the American student nurses told them from outside the door, "You come out of the closet and he is not going to harm you."[18] Amurao and Gargullo also helped another student nurse avoid the tragedy. Neighbor and fellow nurse Tammy Sioukoff had knocked on the rear door of the townhouse in search of some bread for a late-night snack. Speck forced Amurao and Gargullo to go downstairs and open the door, but the Filipino exchange nurses knowingly led him to the front door instead. By that time Sioukoff had left.[19] After Speck had tied up each of the student nurses and then led his first victim out of the room, the Filipino exchange nurses tried to convince the others to fight Speck. They pointed out that Speck had forced his way into their home, that he was armed with a gun and knife, and that he had bound all of them. However, Amurao related that the American student nurses disagreed and talked them out of a collective attempt at resistance: "They told us we more or less had to trust him. Maybe if we are calm and quiet he will be, too. He has been talking to us all and he seems calm enough and that is a good sign."[20]

However, few U.S. news reports highlighted the fighting spirit of the

Filipino exchange nurses. When Pasion and Gargullo were mentioned, it was often in reference to the U.S. Exchange Visitor Program, which the U.S. media portrayed in a positive light as a program that enabled Gargullo and Pasion "to enter a new culture, make new friends, and enjoy the experiences of living in the United States."[21] Hospital exploitation and other abuses of the program were not mentioned. Instead, news reports claimed that the program was mutually beneficial because it enabled Filipino exchange nurses to improve their education as well as helped alleviate U.S. nursing shortages.[22] The Philippine press similarly romanticized the program's educational objectives and the intellectual drive of its Filipino participants. An editorial in the *Philippine Journal of Nursing* honored Gargullo and Pasion as "martyrs to a cause" and contextualized their deaths as occurring "in line of duty." It emphasized that "Filipinos are known far and wide for their passion for education and this can properly be said of the two young nurses, who, not content with their training in the homeland, went to the United States to further their education and enrich their experience with their chosen profession."[23]

Although Speck's victims came from different countries, they were united in the profession of nursing, in the training of South Chicago Community Hospital, in the daily living of their nursing residence, and in the tragedy of the massacre. The U.S. media portrayed the Filipino and American student nurses as friends. The *New York Times* published a photo of Valentina Pasion smiling and conversing with four of the white American student nurses shortly before the massacre.[24] Another photo portrayed the grief of white American nurses after services were held for the two Filipino victims.[25] The terror-stricken words of Amurao after finding the bodies of the victims also found their way to print: "My *friends* are all dead, all dead, all dead. . . . My *friends* are all dead."[26]

The deaths of two Filipino participants in the U.S. Exchange Visitor Program placed the Speck massacre in an international political spotlight. The tragedy connected Filipinos in the Philippines with Americans and Filipinos in the United States. President Johnson contacted President Marcos and asked him to send his condolences to the victims' families. Money was raised on both sides of the ocean for the families of Gargullo and Pasion. The Philippine Nurses Association and its overseas chapter, the PNA of Chicago, raised several thousand dollars for the parents of the two victims; President Ferdinand and First Lady Imelda

Marcos made a personal donation. Philippine and American officials coordinated efforts to honor both the American and Filipino victims. A former Philippine ambassador to the United States worked with the executive director of South Chicago Community Hospital to establish an annual recognition reward for an outstanding exchange nurse from the Philippines in memory of the Filipino victims. The Filipino Students Catholic Association of Chicago requested a requiem mass for all of the victims at the Holy Trinity Catholic Church. The South Chicago Community Hospital also paid tribute to both American and Filipino victims with certificates at the graduation exercises. The theme of the ceremony was "We loved them in life, let us not forget them in death."[27]

THE STAR WITNESS, BUT A SPECK SENSATION

After the massacre, lone survivor Corazon Amurao emerged as the star witness in the case against Richard Speck. Although Amurao suffered from shock immediately after the massacre, soon she was able to give details of Speck's description to a police artist during a two-hour interview. The artist's sketch eventually led to a gas station attendant's recognition of Speck as a seaman seeking work at the nearby National Maritime Union. Police discovered Speck's name on a job application. As Speck had had several jobs as a seaman, his photograph had been filed with the U.S. Coast Guard. Amurao then identified Speck as the intruder from over one hundred photographs of men registered with the U.S. Coast Guard. Her identification set in motion a number of events that led to the location of his whereabouts and his arrest. Amurao was then able to personally identify him in a prison hospital.

Amurao's status as the star witness combined with the American public's fascination with mass murder and bodily violence to make her into a celebrity. Soon after the crime, Amurao appeared in the society pages of the *Chicago Tribune,* leading the gossip column by Herb Lyon, who mused, "Was or wasn't that surviving nurse, Corazon Amurao, lunching at the Sherman's Celtic room with Philippine consul General Provido? At any rate, there'll be no exclusive story sale to any national mag. by courageous Amurao."[28] Amurao's photo appeared next to the column, which then continued to divulge more celebrity sightings of and gossip about Frank Sinatra and Dean Martin. American mainstream magazines

Life and the *Saturday Evening Post* competed for photographs of Amurao and exclusive rights to her story about the night of the massacre. The *Post*'s reported offer of $25,000 for her story was a newsworthy sum at the time.[29] Unlike the Philippine and American lawyers who argued about the potential profits from her story, Amurao rejected these offers, claiming that such publicity tainted the memory of the victims. However, the *Post* paid for Amurao's mother's flight from the Philippines and a writer from the magazine accompanied the mother from the airport. *Life* had also offered to pay the plane fare, but only in exchange for exclusive rights to photographs of the mother and daughter greeting each other at the airport.

The consistency of Amurao's identification of Speck through police interviews and photographs climaxed with her identification of him in court. Amurao's modest physical appearance and demeanor during the prosecution's three-hour direct examination made her the perfect prosecution witness. In the nonfiction book *Born to Raise Hell,* authors Jack Altman and Marvin Ziporyn described the courtroom drama of Amurao's identification of Speck in slow motion with visual and emotional detail:

> The young, bespectacled prosecution counsel gripped the sides of his wooden lectern, his knuckles showing white as he asked in a dry, metallic voice: "Now, Miss Amurao, if you see that same man in the courtroom today who came to your bedroom door on Wednesday night, July 13, 1966, would you please step down and point him out."
>
> It was the time-honored question of all classic murder trials. In the trial of the people of Illinois versus Richard Franklin Speck, the question bore practically the whole burden of the prosecution's case. Now the question was addressed to the sole survivor of a night of mass murder for which endless retelling had rendered the word "horror" most horribly superfluous. Corazon Amurao, the Filipino nurse from San Luis, Batangas, stared intently and unflinchingly at William Martin as he asked the question. Without any word of acknowledgment, she rose slowly as a bailiff opened the gate of the witness stand. In a starched white short-sleeved blouse, dark blue culottes modestly reaching to below the knees of her black-stockinged legs, and flat brown shoes, she walked a dozen short steps to the polished oak defense table. Clutching a white handkerchief in her left fist, she held her tiny four-foot-ten frame erect and steadily raised her right hand to within six inches of Richard Speck's ashen face. "This is the man."

Her small features remained expressionless as her accusing hand hovered by Speck's left cheek a split second longer following her statement. Her four words seemed similarly to hover in the air for that hushed split second.[30]

This moment reconfirmed why Amurao had become an American celebrity. The "time-honored question of all classic murder trials" had been directed toward her. And her statement, "This is the man," was the key element in the American people's case against Speck, perpetrator of the crime of the century.

This description also illustrated the significance of Amurao's modest physical appearance and demeanor. She may have been from San Luis Batangas, but this only added an exotic touch to a description of a beautiful caregiver whose sexual attractiveness had been tempered by her proper woman's attire of a starched blouse, below-the-knee culottes, and flat shoes. Her demeanor was stereotypically female, given her emotional, tearful state. But it was balanced by her steadfastness. Her manner was "highly charged with emotion" but "at once determined." She was "businesslike . . . but not cold and dehumanized." Amurao would break down and weep but then regain "a firm hold on her feelings." Above all was the "sureness of her account of the events," a sureness that was derived from her body language, the way she stared intently and unflinchingly, held her tiny frame "erect," and raised her hand "steadily" to point at Speck's face. Amurao's demeanor reflected that of the ideal nurse, one who could care physically and emotionally for patients in the most trying of times and at the same time remain firm and in control.[31]

In addition to her professional background, Amurao's exotic features fascinated the American press in ways that made her testimony more credible and appealing. Although a *New York Times* article described her speech as "unsophisticated, heavy English," a front-page *Chicago Tribune* article described Amurao's "clear girlish voice" as "tinged with the soft Spanish accent of the tiny Filipino nurse."[32] This article continued to describe Amurao's "small-featured, moon-shaped face" and "the depths of her jet black eyes."[33] Girlish, tiny, and small were among the many adjectives that the press used and that conjured images of an exotic, almost primitive, innocence, an innocence that seemed incapable of falsehood. A front-page *Chicago Daily News* article characterized Amurao as "the beautiful Filipino nurse . . . barely over 5 feet tall and small-boned

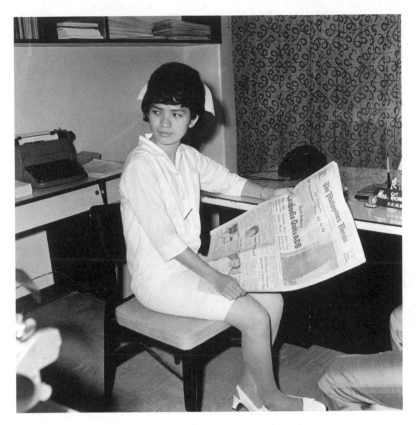

Corazon Amurao, lone survivor of the 1966 Richard Speck massacre in Chicago, reading a newspaper account of her plan to run for councilor in her home town of San Luis, Batangas in the Philippines. From Bettmann/ CORBIS.

with clear fresh skin and glowing dark eyes. . . . Her English, with the Filipino accent, sounds very formal."[34] Confirming Amurao's star qualities, another article presented her as "the delicate Filipino girl" who, "in a day and age when macabre murder trials clog every TV screen . . . projected more vividly than any Oscar winner ever did."[35]

Although Amurao along with the families of the eight slain nurses sued the South Chicago Community Hospital in 1967 for breaching its "custodial" responsibility for the nurses' safety, and settled out of court for an undisclosed figure, Amurao refused to capitalize on the tragedies of others in the press. Decades after the massacre, despite the continuing interest in her story about that night of horror, she refused to be interviewed for retrospectives of the Speck massacre, such as the 1986 special *Chicago Tribune Sunday Magazine* issue devoted to the twentieth anniversary of the massacre.[36] Her final response to the tragedy was to move on with her life, returning to a hero's welcome in the Philippines, working as a nurse at Manila's Far Eastern University Hospital, successfully running for councilor in her hometown of San Luis, Batangas, marrying Bert Atienza (a Filipino lawyer and real estate broker), and raising two children. She eventually returned to the United States. According to a 1992 *Filipino Reporter* article, Corazon Amurao-Atienza worked as a nurse at Georgetown University Hospital in Washington, D.C.[37]

However, Amurao is not remembered for her life after July 14, 1966; rather, she continues to be regarded in an almost mythical way for surviving the massacre. In my interviews, several Filipino nurses expressed admiration for Amurao because she used her wits and will to survive the massacre. The image of Amurao rolling under one of the bunks to evade Speck was the most vivid memory they had of the tragedy. Anita Ramos Nanadiego had just finished her nursing training at Marian School of Nursing in Manila at the time of the massacre. She related, "We were so proud when we heard that it was the Filipino nurse that thought of the right thing to do. In terms of crisis, she was able to deal with that problem."[38]

Although Amurao's evasion of Speck continues to inspire admiration and a fighting spirit among Filipinos and others, her mythical status has also been used in ways that have produced some troubling effects. For example, in Dwight Okita's play, *Richard Speck,* an unnamed Asian American woman recalls being in second grade when the massacre occurred. In her childhood history, the massacre functions as a pivotal moment in her awareness of the violence men commit against women, an awareness that shatters the innocence of her childhood: "I think I was too shy to ask anyone what was going on, so I went to the park behind the building and played on the swings. That night, my parents told me what happened, there were pictures of the bodies on the news. 'He could've stopped at ANY house,' they said." However, rather than send her to the depths of despair and paranoia, the massacre becomes a personal source of strength because of Amurao's story. In the play, the Asian American woman continues: "I always think about that one Filipino nurse who escaped. She hid under the bed. See, that's what I would do. She wanted to save ALL of them. 'There are nine of us, we can take him!' she said. But they were too afraid, so she crawled under the bed—and she lived. I LOVE that—when people trust their instincts." At the end of the play, this personal source of strength is transformed into racial pride as the woman tells the audience: "Those women he killed, they weren't just nurses, you know—they were Asian Americans. Most people don't think about that, but I do. Last May, for Asian American Heritage Month, I made a toast to the nurse that got away—to her courage, her wisdom, her survival."[39]

On one level, the play functions as an important alternative reading to the Speck massacre, one that does not wallow in the senselessness of the crime or in the mainstream American public's obsession with the mass murderer, but rather celebrates the courage, wisdom, and survival of Amurao in the context of racialized consciousness and pride. Ironically, however, Corazon Amurao's name, like that of the Asian American woman character, is never mentioned in the play. The audience comes to know her only as the "Filipino nurse who escaped." Although this act of unnaming was surely intentional—a move that reinforces that the character and the "Filipino nurse who escaped" are both Asian American—the erasure of Amurao's name and the foregrounding of Speck's name in the title of the play both reflect and continue to reinscribe America's pathological public sphere, its obsession over Speck. Erased are the efforts of Merlita Gargullo and Valentina Pasion to resist Speck as well as Amurao's life history. As the Asian American woman in the play rhetorically asks the audience, "You remember, Richard, don't you?"[40]

Amurao may have been the one who escaped and became the prosecution's star witness, but history revealed Speck to be the enduring American celebrity. One year after the massacre, freelance writer Jack Altman and Cook County Hospital staff psychiatrist Martin Ziporyn wrote *Born to Raise Hell: The Untold Story of Richard Speck,* a book that focused on the relationship between Speck and Ziporyn. An excerpt of the book became a cover story for the *Saturday Evening Post*'s July 1, 1967 issue, marking the one-year anniversary of the mass murder. The headline of the issue read: "Inside the Mind of a Murderer: Richard Speck Talks." Underneath, the headline continued: "8 Student Nurses Slain." The cover photograph featured a close-up of Speck's face, with small, wallet-size headshots of his eight victims lined in two rows across his forehead. Although the name of the victim accompanied each of the headshots, the *Post* cover illustrated the American public's growing fascination with the life and mind of murderer Speck and its fading interest in the lives of the young women slain. In such depictions, these women had become only figments of a larger, seemingly more important story about a criminal mind.

Born to Raise Hell promoted and exploited this fascination with Speck by focusing on the complexity of his life story and its relevance for the American mainstream public, a public treated throughout the text as a universal norm. In the text, psychiatrist Ziporyn argues that although Speck was portrayed as a monster in the press, he was essentially a "normal man" whose impulses were "no different" from Ziporyn's own "or anyone else's" for that matter. Although Ziporyn did not deny Speck's murderous actions, he claimed that Speck's behavior was both reflective of his environment and typical of a person with a "brain-damaged personality." The treatment of Speck's life history in the book exemplified what Mark Seltzer has observed to be a foundational script for serial killers, namely, an abusive childhood.[41] In *Born to Raise Hell,* Speck's painful loss of his father as a result of his parents' troubled divorce, his upbringing by his mother and an uncaring stepfather, and his own failed marriage led to a life of alcohol and drugs. Given Speck's background and his series of head injuries, Ziporyn diagnosed Speck as an "obsessive-compulsive individual."[42]

Throughout the text Ziporyn negotiates his analysis of Speck as a personality type that can be categorized and analyzed through the science of psychiatry, with his depiction of Speck as an individual human being. In the end, both analyses conjure a sympathetic portrayal of Speck. By categorizing Speck as a personality type created by an imperfect world, Ziporyn absolves him of blame for his actions: "Like every other human being, you Richard, are the product of your heredity and your environment. You didn't pick either one. I can find what you did terrible. . . . But I can't find you responsible for your actions. . . . You have real brain damage. . . . It's not your fault that you didn't get medical care."[43]

Speck's emotional and childlike behavior invoked pity from the readers. He suffered from depression and suicidal tendencies; he shed tears before his psychiatrist. He claimed that he was "glad" that Corazon Amurao had survived the massacre. He expressed deep sadness for "hurting" and "shaming" his family through his violent actions. He longed for the presence of his real father and suffered from the lack of affection from his stepfather.[44]

Speck's negative experiences with women cast his misogyny in a different light and provided a context for explaining his violence against the student nurses. Readers learned that his wife, Shirley, had been unfaithful to him, and that Gloria Davy, one of the student nurse victims, was a Shirley look-alike. A previous encounter with another woman resulted in Speck's contracting syphilis and subsequently becoming sterile. The racial identity of the woman raised questions about Speck's hatred of Asian women in particular. Speck claimed, "Never forget her. Sure would like to get back at her. She was Chinese or Japanese—some kind of Oriental, know what I mean?"[45]

Through this use of "know what I mean" to refer to the cruelty that all women of color are capable of inflicting on men, *Born to Raise Hell* targeted a heterosexual male readership that on one level bonded with Speck by empathizing with the "dangers" of women, and on another level admired Speck for his newly found sex-symbol stardom. The book describes how a woman named Lois repeatedly wrote letters of support to Speck, included her photo in one of them, and signed her letters "with love." Speck's appeal was transnational. He received a Valentine card from a sixteen-year-old girl in Cebu City, Philippines, describing herself as "one who cares."[46]

Ziporyn used the heterosexist objectification of women to develop his relationship with Speck. In his prison cell, Speck hung a poster of a young woman dressed only in undergarments, which he labeled, "Miss Death Row, U.S.A." He explained to Ziporyn that the poster "brightens up the place," and Ziporyn agreed that there is "nothing like a dame." Ziporyn also employed the public's voyeuristic fascination with sex and violence to raise Speck above the depths of despair. Ziporyn encouraged him, "Half the people think you raped those girls. . . . They think you're the stud of the century. . . . They think you are some kind of sex symbol. Why do you think those women keep writing to you?"[47]

Finally, Speck's individuality—his sex appeal, sense of humor, loyalty to his family, and new interest in painting—hinted at redemption and hope. During his visits with Speck, Ziporyn gave him presents, particularly painting sets, upon discovering that Speck enjoyed the activity. During one visit, Ziporyn attempted to instill in Speck the will to live by referring to what he had still to offer society: "You still have something to give. You have real artistic ability."[48]

While newspapers published Speck's amateur attempts at painting horses, creative writing presented an alternative reading of the sensation over Speck.[49] In Lawson Fusao Inada's 1971 poem "Bandstand," Inada played on mainstream America's glorification of youth and sex. The title conjured images of Dick Clark's all-American classic show *American Bandstand,* with its young participants, trendy dances, and sexual energy. The poem opened "innocently" enough this way:

> The focus is youth—casual
> stances on the ballroom floor.
>
> The boys are smooth; the girls
> stick out all over.
>
> Every mother's son
> calls the tune
> and bodies snap into action,
>
> slanting the best angles to the camera.
>
> They have been carefully screened.
>
> Outside, the dusk on Philadelphia . . .
>
> Meanwhile, they reach their peak,
> doing "The Hitchhiker" on national TV—
> standing in place, thumbing a ride . . .

These opening stanzas and the sexually enticing but still good-old-American-fun images that they produce are shattered as Inada continues:

> One of them, of course,
> is Richard Speck—
>
> he's in the corner of your screen—
>
> having a blast,
> dancing his ass off
> with a teased little trick.
>
> He got here early,
> stashed his Mustang in the alley;

he'll probably get tagged
but who cares? —

He's got a part-time gig.
She finally accepted.
He's on the scene.

Then it's time for an ad —
some huge tube oozing out of itself . . .

And ol' Dickie, cool
gum-popping Dickie,
struts it into the men's room

for a smoke, to contemplate
a pimple, to ponder whether to get a new
tattoo and join the Merchant Marines,
for kicks —

then makes it on out to join the music.[50]

The mention of Speck's name in the context of an American bandstand powerfully disrupts the typically American, seemingly innocent images conjured at the beginning of the poem. This jarring effect, combined with Inada's insistence that "one of them, *of course,* is Richard Speck," plays on and critiques average Americans' shock about the massacre as well as their fascination over "cool, gum-popping Dickie," also known as mass murderer Speck. The poem suggests that such violence is nurtured by an American culture that commodifies and then sells sex for a male audience: "then it's time for an ad — some huge tube oozing out of itself." However, mainstream America's mistaken beliefs in its youthful innocence renders this violence an abhorrent anomaly. In addition, Inada's racialized identity as a Japanese American and an important writer of the Asian American movement — a movement greatly inspired and informed by African American, American Indian, and Chicano civil rights movements — implies that the poem also critiques mainstream America's racialized belief in white American innocence and its displacement of the cause of violence onto the bodies of Americans of color, bodies coded in the Chicago press as "street mobs" and "civil rights spokesmen."[51]

While these alternative readings of the Speck sensation powerfully critique the narratives publicized in Altman and Ziporyn's book, the book is significant because it is a testimony of Richard Speck's long-lasting popularity. Speck was and continues to be an American cultural phenomenon. *Born to Raise Hell: The Untold Story of Richard Speck,* first published by Grove Press in 1967, was reprinted by Hallberg Publishing Corporation in 1984, almost two decades after the massacre that catapulted Speck to fame, and retitled *Speck: The Untold Story of a Mass Murderer.* Although the body of the text is identical in both editions, several changes in the new edition indicate the level of Speck's growing stardom. In *Born to Raise Hell,* a photograph of Corazon Amurao, with her arm intertwined with that of her mother and followed by a detective as she leaves the trial, was placed at the end of the text. Amurao's mother is looking down, and her hand is tightly clasping a handkerchief or tissue. By contrast, Corazon Amurao looks straight ahead of her, head held high. She appears calm, yet determined, her eyes staring intently and unflinchingly before her, like the description of her demeanor in the courtroom. This final photograph and the title, *Born to Raise Hell,* a reference to both the phrase tattooed on Speck's arm and the heinous nature of his crimes, conjure memories of the massacre, the dead, and the survivor. In the 1984 reprint, this photograph was removed from the text. The name "Speck" was edited from the subtitle and featured in the main title.

In the 1984 reprint of *Speck,* a new introduction written by Thomas M. Gannon, director of the Woodstock Theological Seminary of Georgetown University, characterizes the book as "a praiseworthy contribution to the understanding of murder."[52] The back cover includes excerpts from reviews in the *New York Times Book Review, Library Journal,* and *Newsweek* that also endorse Altman and Ziporyn's book. Anthony Boucher of the *New York Times Book Review* commends Ziporyn's work as "so skillful." Allan Angoff of the *Library Journal* characterizes *Speck* as a story for scientific and academic experts — "the pathologist, criminologist, and sociologist" — as well as laypersons. S. K. Oberback of *Newsweek* likens Speck's story to those of "thousands of criminals" with "a lamentable story of growing up askew."

Born to Raise Hell and its reprint as *Speck,* reviewers' endorsements of the book as "imperative reading," the growing marginalization of the memory of the victims, and the rising celebrity status of Speck reveal the ways American society grappled with the Speck massacre. Initially denounced by some and glorified by others, Speck became an individual who was to be understood, not stereotyped, and pitied, not damned. Regardless of what you thought of him, Speck was important. Such fascination with Richard Speck—as an American individual, criminal type, and cultural icon—was a racialized and gendered privilege that would not be bestowed on two Filipino immigrant nurses accused of murder.

THE TRIALS OF FILIPINA NARCISO AND LEONORA PEREZ

Between July and August 1975, up to thirty-five patients suffered from respiratory arrest at the VA Hospital in Ann Arbor, Michigan, and some of these patients died.[53] Although VA Hospital officials initially denied any criminal wrongdoing, the number of breathing failures significantly exceeded the monthly average rates. Because the VA is a federal institution, the FBI launched an investigation and eventually accused two Filipino nurses, Filipina Narciso and Leonora Perez, of committing the crimes. In June 1976, Narciso and Perez were arrested and indicted on ten counts of poisoning, five counts of murder, and one count of conspiracy.

At the time of her arrest, Narciso was a thirty-year-old permanent resident who had applied for U.S. citizenship. She arrived in the United States from the Philippines in May 1971 and worked as a registered nurse at University of Alabama Hospital before she began working at the VA in Ann Arbor in November 1972. Perez was a thirty-one-year-old permanent resident who had also applied for U.S. citizenship. She arrived in the United States from the Philippines in March 1971. At the time of her arrest, Perez was married to Epifanio Perez Jr., who was also a permanent resident, and they had a three-year-old son, Christopher. Perez was also four months pregnant. Neither Narciso nor Perez had a criminal record and, during the initial stages of the investigation, they cooperated with the investigation by testifying before a grand jury on two occasions and appearing in a line-up.

Assistant U.S. Attorney Richard Delonis admitted from the beginning of the investigation that the case was highly circumstantial because of the absence of evidence—murder weapon, direct eyewitness testimonies, confessions, and fingerprints—traditionally used to convict criminals. Yet, the government's strong motivations for solving the case of the VA murders and its use of seemingly unlimited resources of money and staff helped shape a powerful case against Narciso and Perez. The VA murders case came at a time when it was important for the U.S. government, and specifically the FBI, to win. In April 1975, America lost the war in Vietnam to communists. The mood in America about the Vietnam War began with optimism, patriotism, and confidence but ended with disillusionment and humiliation by a tenacious Southeast Asian people. Also at this time, the FBI was investigating cases involving Patty Hearst and Jimmy Hoffa, both unsuccessfully. Winning a high-profile case, such as the VA murders, could redeem the government and the agency.[54]

The extensive resources — time, staff, and money — used by the FBI in its investigation reflected its strong commitment to solve the case. As defense attorney Thomas O'Brien observed, "When the Federal Bureau of Investigation goes to work, it can be impressive. They did not just come to visit — they moved in."[55] The agency established a field headquarters in the hospital, initially on the ground floor, and then relocated to a larger area on the fifth floor. In its seven-week occupation of the hospital, approximately twenty FBI agents conducted interviews with the hospital's seven hundred full-time employees. Special telephone lines had been installed and "volumes of interview material assembled by agents remain[ed] under lock and key."[56] Furthermore, the agency deployed hundreds of agents nationwide to interview former employees of the hospital. Defense attorneys for Narciso and Perez estimated that at various times, more than two hundred FBI agents and employees worked on the case and that the FBI spent over $1 million for the investigation.

As the agency's investigation intensified, Narciso, Perez, and other VA nurses accused the FBI of harassment. The FBI interrogated Narciso three times and Perez four times in August 1975, and then interrogated each of them one more time in September. After her fourth interrogation, some of Narciso's coworkers found her huddled and shaking in a corner unable to function. Agents had allegedly made references to her religious beliefs. These interrogations led Narciso and Perez to seek counsel in early October 1975.

Narciso told her lawyer that after a six-hour interrogation, the FBI agent warned her, "Watch the line on this piece of paper. This is your life up to now. You have been happy. You have made friends. You have been successful in your profession. Now your life is over. I know you are a religious person. You had better light a candle for yourself."[57] According to Narciso, the agent drew her picture repeatedly and commented several times that she was only twenty-nine years old. Agents also intimidated Perez by saying that she had "better be prepared to say good-bye to her family."[58]

The FBI denied charges of harassment and overzealousness. Agents claimed that Narciso had been calm and composed throughout the interrogation. Whereas a combination of steadfastness and emotional breakdown had strengthened Amurao's credibility as a witness, U.S. attorneys associated Narciso's changing emotional states with criminality: "[Narciso's] later appearance of being upset could be attributed to . . . fabrication [or] to feelings of guilt." The government then characterized both Narciso and Perez's allegations of harassment as "selective distortions of fact to apparently deliberate disregard for truth."[59]

Aside from its own agents, the FBI invested a significant amount of its resources to employ numerous scientific, medical, and psychological experts, who, before and during the trial, constructed the "facts" of the crimes and a profile of the perpetrator(s). The FBI relied heavily on psychiatric profiles to narrow its search, working with psychiatrists, such as Derek H. Miller and David Abrahamson, who were experts in crime and homicide. The authority of these professionals grounded a complex, highly circumstantial, and politically charged case with rationality, order, and objectivity.

The U.S. attorneys explained, "The keystone to putting the government's proofs in a full and proper perspective is a comprehensive understanding of the operative medical-scientific evidence thus far adduced at trial."[60] According to the government, this understanding involved four main points. First, the respiratory arrests of the patients were medically unexpected. Second, the administration of a muscle-relaxant drug precipitated these respiratory arrests. Third, the drug pancuronium bromide (the basic active ingredient of Pavulon) was present in the urine, lung, and liver tissue specimens of the victims. The fourth, and perhaps most significant, point was that the Pavulon used in these crimes had to have been administered in a rapid fashion as opposed to slow infusion. Thus, U.S. attorneys argued that Pavulon had to have been administered to victim John McCreary less than three minutes before he was discovered suffering from a respiratory arrest. U.S. attorneys used the testimony of the victims' attending physicians, pulmonary medical specialists, anesthesiologists, forensic chemists, and forensic pathologists to support each of these points.

Given this understanding of the crimes, U.S. attorneys then highlighted the repeated presence of Narciso and/or Perez at the bedside of victims Charles Gasmire, John McCreary, and William Loesch a few minutes before their arrest. They concluded that when these circumstances of repeated presence were taken together, they rose above the status of inexplicable coincidence and signified criminal intent and activity. Although eyewitness testimonies on several counts placed only either Narciso or Perez at individual crime scenes, U.S. attorneys argued that the crimes were so identical that Narciso and Perez "had to be in criminal concert."[61]

The defense attempted to undermine the government's case in multiple ways. First, they cast doubt on the U.S. attorneys' scientific and medical construction of the crimes. The defense highlighted alternative ways in which Pavulon could have been administered through the intravenous bags of victim-patients, suggesting that the injection of the drug need not have occurred only a few minutes before the arrests. They questioned the sterility and safety of the IV bags used by the VA Hospital during the summer of 1975 after a section of Baxter-Travenol Laboratory, the sole provider of the intravenous fluids and additive fluids for the hospital, had closed down during the time of the respiratory arrests. The defense also emphasized that some of the respiratory arrests discussed in the prosecution's case had not been recorded in the victims' medical records, suggesting that these records were incomplete or had been tampered with.

Second, the defense challenged the government's theory about Narciso and Perez's act of conspiracy by revealing that the defendants had known each other for only three to four weeks before the series of respiratory arrests occurred. They met for the first time when they were both assigned to the intensive care units in the spring of 1975. They did not socialize after work and they were not close friends—until the pressures of the FBI investigation pushed them closer together.

Third, the defense disputed the government's association of Narciso and Perez's repeated presence near the victims shortly before their arrest with criminality. They emphasized that none of the eyewitnesses saw Narciso or Perez with a syringe filled with Pavulon, nor did they observe the defendants injecting the drug in the IV tubing of the victims. The

defense pointed out that Narciso and Perez were registered nurses working in the intensive care units where the respiratory arrests had taken
place, and thus their presence in these areas was a part of their nursing
duties. As Perez claimed after the trial, "Our mere presence at the bedside
of patients shouldn't convict us. It was our job."[62] According to the
defense, the connection between their professional presence near the
victims and criminal activity involved too many inferences. For example,
in the case of victim Charles Gasmire, they noted:

> Richard Gasmire testified that he observed Mrs. Perez standing by his
> father's bed during the one minute preceding his father's arrest. . . . Rich-
> ard Gasmire did not see Mrs. Perez with a syringe or administering any
> medication to his father. Moreover, no testimony was introduced to show
> that Pavulon, or any syringes, were found in Gasmire's room, or in any
> way connected with Mrs. Perez. . . . From the mere fact of Mrs. Perez'
> presence in Mr. Gasmire's room, one must infer that she was there for the
> purpose of administering medication, that the medication included Pavu-
> lon, and from all of these inferences, to infer that she intended to injure
> Mr. Gasmire. Such piling of inferences upon inferences is clearly unjusti-
> fiable and impermissible.[63]

Finally, the defense challenged the government's use of eyewitness
testimony in two ways: by revealing that eyewitnesses had seen several
persons near the victims shortly before their respiratory arrest and by
casting doubt on the credibility of some of the prosecution's key eyewitnesses. For example, survivor-victim McCreary identified several persons
as his assailants, including a Caucasian woman (who had been granted
immunity by the prosecution for testifying before the grand jury), a
Mexican female, and a Mexican male.[64] The defense accused the prosecution of using eyewitness testimony selectively, for example by deleting
McCreary's reference to a Mexican male as his assailant in three interviews conducted by an FBI intern. The mother of victim Loesch testified
that she had seen a "man in a green scrubsuit" enter her son's room
shortly before his respiratory arrest.[65]

Richard Neely was a particularly important eyewitness for the government's case as he was the first person to identify "a Filipino girl" before
his respiratory arrest, whom he later identified as Leonora Perez. Until
his identification of Perez, the government's case had focused solely on
Narciso. The defense attacked the credibility of Neely because he suf-

fered from memory loss and alcoholism. During a cross-examination by the defense, Neely lamented, "I was disgusted with myself because I couldn't remember everybody I met at the hospital."[66] Neely admitted to drinking fifteen to twenty-five beers daily from morning to night and to suffering complete memory loss after drinking.

The defense also attempted to reveal Neely's biases in favor of the FBI and against Perez. During cross-examination, when defense attorney Burgess asked Neely what he thought of the FBI, Neely responded, "I think they're a wonderful organization, and they do wonders for America." By contrast, Neely described Perez as a "cold, professional person" who "was more of a lady that just thought of business . . . hospital and nurse business."[67]

Furthermore, the defense revealed that Neely's identification of a "Filipino girl" as his assailant was questionable because Neely was unable to distinguish Filipinos from Japanese, Chinese, and other Asians. All Asians essentially looked alike to him. In the cross-examination about Neely's sessions with a psychiatrist, Dr. Ging, Neely attempted to describe her race and national origin with much confusion:

Defense: Mr. Neely, did you see this Dr. Ging, the psychiatrist . . . ? Do you want to describe what she looks like?

Neely: Pleasant little old lady. . . .

Defense: Was she — is she Caucasian?

Neely: Rather, yeah.

Defense: Was she white, Mr. Neely? Was she black? Was she Oriental?

Neely: Possibly a little Oriental. . . .

Defense: Do you know whether or not she was Japanese, Chinese, or Filipino?

Neely: No, I didn't ask her. . . .

Defense: You're not able to do that, huh? Able to tell, whether or not someone is Japanese, Chinese, or Filipino?

Neely: To a certain extent, yes.

Defense: All right. Using those abilities that you have, do you have any better recollection as to if she falls into one of those categories?

Neely: My guess would have been Filipino.

Defense: Okay. Why do you guess that?

Neely: Because she was so nice.

Defense: All right. I see. Filipinos are nice?

Neely: Yes.

Defense: As distinguished from Japanese and Chinese? They're not nice. Is that what you're saying to us?

Neely: They're nice too. . . . He [*sic*] looked rather—a little Filipino to me.

Defense: . . . What does that mean? . . . How is she different from a Japanese?

Neely: I wouldn't know exactly, how to distinguish her exactly from a Japanese.

Defense: Okay. Do you know how to distinguish her from a Chinese?

Neely: No. She could have been possibly.

Defense: Okay. So you don't really know what she was?

Neely: Oh, no. No. No, I don't exactly know what she was. No.[68]

In later testimony, Neely revealed that although he had fought in the Philippines during World War II and although he remembered that Filipinos "were all for America," he could not really distinguish Japanese from Filipinos because "they have resemblances that are similar."[69]

THE ENIGMA OF THE LITTLE FILIPINO

Such seemingly positive stereotypes of Filipinos as "so nice" and "all for America" may have contributed to the optimism of the defense at the beginning of the case. Defense lawyer Thomas O'Brien claimed, "The best thing we [the defense] have going in the case is Filipina Narciso and Leonora Perez. Once the jury has the chance to see and hear them, there won't be any questions in their minds either."[70] O'Brien believed that Narciso and Perez "looked innocent" and noted that news accounts described them as "pleasant, open, polite."[71] Even the prosecuting attorneys admitted that it would be difficult to prove that Narciso and Perez—"small, soft-spoken, young women"—could be involved in such a crime.[72]

However, these positive images of Narciso and Perez coexisted with negative ones conjured by news media, a popular nonfiction book, and the prosecution's questions and statements. Narciso and Perez's gender, race, and national origin could invoke multiple and conflicting meanings. One could also imagine these nice, small, soft-spoken Filipino women to be women who poisoned, inscrutable Orientals and savage natives.

The FBI investigation of the VA murders focused on the nurses of the VA Hospital because psychiatrist and criminal expert Derek Miller, who prepared the profile of the killer, advised the FBI to search for a woman, as poison is a woman's weapon. Given the gendered, women's work of nursing, FBI agents placed the VA nurses under suspicion, and not the doctors. Yet, although the FBI also interrogated and intimidated the white nurses and nursing assistants of the intensive care unit where the poisonings took place, they did not become the government's number one suspects, even in the case of white American nursing supervisor Betty Jakim. On March 13, 1977, midway through jury selection, the *Detroit Free Press* reported that Jakim had confessed to her psychiatrist before her suicide on February 3 that she was responsible for the deaths. She also left a note insisting that Narciso and Perez were innocent. Jakim reportedly suffered from severe depression and was at one point confined for a time in an Ann Arbor mental hospital. However, her psychiatrist refused to comment on her case. And when the attorneys for Narciso and Perez attempted to obtain Jakim's psychiatric records, they had been placed under a protective order. One week after summarizing the findings from the *Detroit Free Press,* the *New York Times* reported that although Jakim was taking cancer-fighting drugs that could alter perception, she was an excellent nurse who "really cared about patients" and who "was very qualified, very skilled."[73]

While the selfless image of the nurse may have made such crimes against her patients seem unthinkable, the stereotype of the inscrutable Oriental — a sneaky and sinister, indistinguishable Asiatic being — applied to the seemingly soft-spoken Filipino nurses and corroborated Miller's conclusion that the perpetrator(s) of the crimes would have to have been "a very clever fellow."[74] Thus Richard Neely struggled with guilt as he testified against Narciso and Perez — "I shouldn't have said I didn't like them too much" — while at the same time pointing to their ambiguous, suspicious qualities: "Just suspicion . . . I don't know why I should be suspicious of them either."[75]

The image of Narciso and Perez as Filipino versions of Asian stereotypes Fu Manchu and the Dragon Lady appeared in a popular nonfiction book entitled *The Mysterious Deaths at Ann Arbor* published in 1976. Unlike *Born to Raise Hell* and its reprint *Speck,* the vast majority of the 253 pages of text in *The Mysterious Deaths* was devoted to the crimes committed in the VA Hospital as opposed to an up-close and personal look at the alleged perpetrators Narciso and Perez. Filipina Narciso did not appear in the text until page 120. The first 120 pages reconstructed the poisonings and murders committed by "a figure in white, it is now believed," in the VA Hospital. The opening chapters detailed the suffering endured by the victims, elderly U.S. veterans who author Robert Wilcox portrayed as all-American, blue-collar men: "farmers, factory workers, small-town men who spent long hours standing at assembly lines in Detroit auto plants or working small plots of land."[76]

From the beginning of the text, Wilcox made full use of the negative connotations of silence and darkness in describing the "most chilling medical horror story of our time." In the context of the Richard Speck trial, the media described Corazon Amurao as "silent" and "dark," but they also described her as slim and assured, conjuring an image of an attractive, exotic, and smart young woman. In the case of the VA murders, the use of "dark" had a different connotation, a deadly one. In Wilcox's depiction of the murders, he characterized the poisonous injections as "a sinister blackness" that overpowered the victims during "those dark days of July." In his reconstruction of "one of the darkest possibilities" that might have taken place at the VA in the summer of 1975, the perpetrator was a figure who "moves quietly in the dim light" and "goes silently by."[77]

When Filipina Narciso finally appeared In *The Mysterious Deaths,* Wilcox offered his readers both positive and negative images of her. However, these contradictory images were not an attempt at an objective, balanced depiction of Narciso but rather a confirmation of the inscrutability of the Filipino nurse. According to Wilcox, Narciso had a "disarming manner," a "soft voice," a "shy demeanor." She appeared "almost apologetic" and "frequently smiling." Yet, immediately after this "favorable" description, Wilcox continued that "it must have been difficult to picture her cold-bloodedly injecting poison into McCreary's IV. But then again . . . a killer of this sort has got to be insane—perhaps schizophrenic. . . . she easily could be hiding another face."[78]

This "other" face of the inscrutable Oriental explained how someone as disarming, shy, and apologetic as Narciso might also be a cold-blooded murderer. Echoing the dramatic rhetorical strategies of writer Sax Rohmer in his early twentieth-century pulp fiction novels about Fu

Manchu and his sinister plot to take over the world, Wilcox suggested to his readers that "such was the enigma of the little Filipino: responsible, considerate, shy. But was it a veil hiding evil beneath?"[79]

While Wilcox highlighted Oriental inscrutability as a possible explanation for Narciso and Perez's criminal behavior, the nurses' racialized identities as Filipinos offered an additional explanation: native savagery. Unlike Altman and Ziporyn, who detailed Speck's childhood to explain the Chicago massacre, Wilcox pointed to the nurses' national origin and citizenship. Although Wilcox acknowledged that Narciso was a U.S. permanent resident, he emphasized that "in plain language, until [U.S.] citizenship is granted, she is an alien [who] retains her Filipino citizenship." Both Narciso and Perez were from the Philippines, which Wilcox described as, "for the most part, jungly, hot, and steamy," a description that conjured images of savage Filipino natives. And, according to Wilcox, the nature of the VA murders suggested "a real and monstrous savagery in the killer." The image of "jungly" natives committing the murders appeared in the opening chapter, in which Wilcox informed his readers that Pavulon, the poison allegedly used in the crimes, was "a poison derived from special tropical plants and used, for instance, by South American jungle Indians on the tips of darts shot to kill game."[80]

The contemporary U.S. recruitment of Filipino nurses along with the history of America's colonial presence in the Philippines complicated this simplistic vision of Filipino native savagery. Wilcox connected Narciso's motivations for becoming a nurse with U.S. colonialism in the Philippines, specifically its system of hospitals that trained Filipino nurses. He acknowledged that the contemporary U.S. health care system actively recruited Filipino nurses to work in the United States. This market was lucrative for American recruiters, who received "$1,000 a head" for importing Filipino nurses in groups. Wilcox also mentioned the support Narciso received from former VA patients, such as James E. Thayer. Thayer wrote a letter to the *Ann Arbor News,* which weaved praise for Narciso's nursing skills with his World War II reminiscences:

> Two years ago I was in the VA Hospital for a very serious back operation. . . . In that time, I had great doctors and nurses. . . . One of these great and lovely girls was a foreign girl, many miles from her home. But to her, we were the men of the Army, Navy and Marine Corps who fought for, and sustained injury in defense of her country, in freeing that land from the

Japanese. . . . This girl would come to my bedside and ask if I was all right, if I needed anything, light a cigarette for me, get me a glass of water, bathe my forehead and talk with me. Nothing was too great a task. . . . I can only speak for myself, but I feel sure that many of the patients you cared for with compassion and understanding, will join me in a prayer. . . . Good luck, and God bless you . . . P. I. Narciso, R.N.[81]

Thayer's "positive" portrayal of Narciso illustrated one form of the persistence of a culture of U.S. imperialism, the ways in which colonial narratives of U.S. benevolence had been perpetuated as American "defense" and "liberation" of the Philippines in World War II and the postwar period. The "greatness" and "loveliness" of Filipino nurses continued to be inextricably linked to and dependent on these stories of American goodness and heroism.

"The enigma of the little Filipino" referred to these tensions and contradictions surviving from U.S. colonial rule. Narciso and Perez were part of a postcolonial legacy of the American introduction of professional nursing in the islands. According to U.S. colonial narratives of benevolence, American nurses and doctors trained young Filipino women to create a healthy and modern nation, and saved them from continuing their native, dirty, and backward ways. Yet although Filipino nurses earned professional degrees and wore white uniforms, they could still be simultaneously racialized as savage in late twentieth-century America.

A review of *The Mysterious Deaths in Ann Arbor* appeared in the leftist Filipino American publication *Ang Katipunan,* which criticized Wilcox for his racist assumptions, artificial suspense, and irresponsible journalism. According to reviewer Sherry Valparaiso, "It is in the best tradition of the American publishing world to make a fast buck by exploiting the tragedy of others."[82] However, these racialized images of Narciso and Perez as dark, deadly natives were not confined to Wilcox's text, but made their way into mainstream publications, prosecution witness testimony, and the prosecution attorneys' questions and statements in court. For example, mainstream magazines such as *Time* also referred to the drug Pavulon as jungle poison, "the lethal plant toxin used by South American Indians to tip poison darts."[83]

According to prosecution witness Richard Neely, even if Filipino nurses could simultaneously embody the potential for both native savagery as well as for professional medical care, this would not necessarily be a bad thing if they practiced their nursing duties on the right side of the ocean, that being in the Philippines and not the United States. As nurses in the Philippines, they fulfilled American benevolent objectives. Neely's testimony illustrated the "logic" of this contradictory benevolence toward Filipinos. After he claimed that he had attempted to "protect" Perez in the investigation by not promptly identifying her as his assailant, Neely explained his actions this way:

> Neely: You can have feelings for other people. I was in the Philippines during the war and I made lots of friends over there, and I went to their villages. They lived in little villages built on little sticks, posts up, and I saw that they didn't have anything. . . . And why should I hurt one of them and I know she could do a whole — an awful lot of good back there and I didn't want to hurt her because she could do so much good back there. . . .
>
> Defense: This woman who you believed was killing people in the hospital, who you believe tried to kill you, who you didn't like, and you're telling us here that you didn't tell the FBI because you were concerned whether or not she could go back to the Philippines and be a successful nurse? Is that what you're telling us?
>
> Neely: Sure. Exactly. And she could have, if she — if she ever went back there, she could have.
>
> Defense: You didn't want to interrupt those plans, didn't want to send that murderer to jail; right, Mr. Neely? Didn't want to stop that murderer; let her go back to the Philippines?
>
> Neely: You're exactly right.[84]

In choosing to remain on the wrong side of the ocean, nonwhite and dark-skinned Narciso and Perez suffered the consequences of being non-Americans and racialized minorities. Neely, in another display of benevolent guilt as he testified against Perez, said that he "pitied" her and "all Filipino women" as they had two strikes against them for being foreign and dark:

> Defense: Now I think you said that you felt that this one Filipino woman had two strikes against her.
>
> Neely: Not just that one woman. All Filipino women. All foreign people from a foreign country.
>
> Defense: What are those strikes that they would have against them?
>
> Neely: Well, for one thing, being a foreigner from out of the country.

Defense: Yes. Why is that a strike against them?

Neely: Because they ain't American.

Defense: And somehow that makes them not as good in someone's eyes?

Neely: Possibly.

Defense: In your eyes?

Neely: Not mine, no.

Defense: You said there were two strikes against them in your mind and that was one of them. Did you not say that?

Neely: No. I would not — not in my mind. I thought they would have two strikes [against] them according to . . .

Defense: Other things other people [told] you?

Neely: What I had heard and [been] brought up [with] all my life.

Defense: Are you saying that the people that you'd been around and you grew up with had expressed some prejudice for people that came from other countries?

Neely: There had been remarks made like that, yes.

Defense: What was the second strike against her?

Neely: Being dark.

Defense: Being dark?

Neely: Yes.

Defense: And in what way is that a strike against her?

Neely: Colored people have a strike against them right off the bat, for being colored.

Defense: Which color, sir?

Neely: Black.

Defense: There are many colors, are there not?

Neely: Yes.

Defense: All right. You're talking about black people having a strike against them?

Neely: Yes, to a certain extent, yes.[85]

The divisive issues of race and skin color were complex ones that went beyond simple binary categories of black versus white, and by extension "people of color" versus "white people." The discourse of American benevolence — in this case, the narrative of Americans' "protection" of their Filipino "little brown sisters" — divided blacks and Filipinos by ranking them in a racial hierarchy, with Filipinos seemingly above and black people below. At the beginning of his testimony, Neely claimed that he had remembered all along that Perez had been the last person he had seen before his respiratory arrest. Yet, in his "pity" for Perez, he "deliberately" avoided revealing this information to investigators and others at first. He also attempted to protect her by telling investigators and others who questioned him of a mysterious black man: "To get away from talking about her, I would say that there was a colored fellow who used to come into my room an awful lot." Although Neely was unaware of the man's identity and activities, this man displayed no signs of any criminal intent or activity. Yet this black man's presence, according to Neely, became "just enough to give me an excuse or an idea to throw the blame onto him when I was talking to somebody."[86]

Neely, who claimed that one could "have feelings for other people," invoked a racialist ploy of "protecting" Leonora Perez by implicating an innocent black man. His testimony revealed the way one could conflate Filipinos and blacks through their "dark" skin color on the one hand, and then *seemingly* rank Filipinos over blacks through benevolent "protection." I highlight the adverb "seemingly," however, because Neely's protection of Perez was no less racist. With his benevolent fantasies of Perez returning to the Philippines and "doing a whole lot of good" there unfulfilled, Neely labeled Narciso and Perez "a couple of slant-eyed bitches" and claimed that there was a conspiracy of 1,800 Filipino nurses in the United States determined to kill U.S. veterans.[87]

ALIEN OTHERS VERSUS *OUR* ANCESTORS

Although Neely's observations seemed irrational and extreme, U.S. attorneys used the "two strikes" against all Filipino women that Neely had referred to during the bond hearing and the trial. The prosecution attempted to "other" Narciso and Perez through references to their foreign status, emphasizing that they were resident aliens, non–U.S. citizens, and natives of the Philippines. After defense witnesses testified to the professional and good-natured character of both defendants during the bond hearing, the prosecuting attorney began cross-examination by asking the witnesses to clarify Narciso and Perez's "ties to the community." The pattern included questions such as, "Can you tell me how strong Mrs. Perez' ties are to the Detroit or county area surrounding Detroit?" and "Am I correct that you stated that you would not be able to tell this Court the extent of ties of either defendant to the community?"[88]

They also questioned defense witnesses about Narciso's and Perez's relatives living in the Philippines; the majority of Narciso's nine siblings and her parents remained there.

The defense emphasized that Narciso and Perez were U.S. permanent residents and that they had relatives living in the United States. Defense witness Grace Cabaya testified that Narciso had a sister in Alabama, a brother in Chicago, and a sister who lived with her in Ypsilanti, Michigan. However, the prosecution attempted to undermine Narciso's and Perez's American ties vis-à-vis their relatives in the United States by revealing that these relatives were not U.S. citizens themselves. The prosecution also challenged the credibility of Filipino defense witnesses by highlighting their own foreign status. For example, the prosecution opened their cross-examination of Cabaya by asking her about her own citizenship status. Like Narciso and Perez, Cabaya held a U.S. permanent resident visa.

In the prosecuting attorney's opening remarks at the trial, U.S. Assistant Attorney Richard Yanko used the "second strike" of being dark against the defendants by using adjectives that conflated darkness with imminent danger when describing the case of the VA murders. According to Yanko, Narciso and Perez were guilty of "one of history's *darkest* crimes." He claimed that history would be made in the courtroom, "*dark* history, criminal history, history *our ancestors* never willed upon us."[89]

During the trial, the prosecution further highlighted the racialized and foreign background of the defendants by repeatedly juxtaposing their testimonies with those of the white American prosecution eyewitnesses and then questioning Narciso and Perez about who was "really" telling the truth:

> Prosecutor: Up to this time you had been with Mrs. Perez, from the time that you went visiting, correct?
>
> Narciso: Yes.
>
> Prosecutor: And isn't this when Mrs. DeHate saw you alone in the hallway going toward Herman?
>
> Narciso: I did not go back to 5 West.
>
> Prosecutor: Didn't you wave to her?
>
> Narciso: No, I did not.
>
> Prosecutor: Didn't she say that you waved to her?
>
> Narciso: That's what she testified.
>
> Prosecutor: But, she's [Mrs. DeHate's] wrong.[90]

Defense attorney O'Brien objected because the prosecutor was asking the defendant to characterize the accuracy of the prosecution witness. The judge also warned the prosecution that such characterization was the responsibility of the jury. Despite the objection, the prosecutor immediately continued with the same line of questioning. O'Brien objected on at least four more occasions as the cross-examination continued.

Yet, in his closing arguments, Yanko emphasized that the defendants' testimony contradicted the multiple testimonies of American doctors, nurses, war veterans, and their family members. These contradictions translated into the inability of Narciso and Perez to substantiate their innocence. This inability signified guilt. In his final words to the jury before their deliberation, Yanko emphasized a phrase, *"Nemo Dat, Qui Non Habet,"* that he had learned from a law school professor. He concluded that "this catchy phrase perhaps is appropriate at this moment, because it refers to what the Defense is. *Nemo Dat, Qui Non Habet.* He who hath not, cannot give."[91]

AMERICAN NIGHTMARE

In a *Detroit Free Press* interview before the trial commenced, Filipina Narciso characterized her experience as a "nightmare." Leonora Perez revealed the painful ways her husband and son had been affected by the publicity of the case. Her son was "too young" to understand what was happening with the investigation of the murders, but old enough to see his mother's arrest on television. "You can't erase it from his mind," she lamented. As for her husband, "he just cried and cried and shut off the TV."[92] In late 1976, as they awaited trial in their homes, both women had their phones disconnected after receiving harassing phone calls.[93]

The "nightmare" of the FBI investigation, publicity, and upcoming trial led both women to reflect sadly on their romanticization of America while they were still in the Philippines, an idealism created by narratives of America as a land of promise that had been popularized by Filipinos as well as Americans. Narciso's father worked as a civilian for the U.S. Navy. She reminisced, "My father thought highly of the United States. He told me . . . we were liberated by the Americans and they're good people. When we were young, we called them [American servicemen] Joe— Victory Joe." Perez recalled, "When I was a kid, we used to study American history. And I was just fascinated to see the United States and to work here."[94]

However, the day after their convictions, Perez insisted that "[the jury] didn't do the right thing." Although she remained confident about their lawyers, she added, "But I don't know about American justice." Narciso said that she too was "disillusioned" by the American justice system.[95]

One of the greatest hardships Narciso and Perez faced as they prepared their defense was the limited nature of their economic resources in comparison to those of the U.S. government. Both women had been suspended from their jobs after their arrests. With little income, they devoted their time to helping prepare for their defense. According to defense lawyer Thomas O'Brien, Narciso set up an office in her basement and spent ten to twelve hours a day reviewing medical records. She explained, "I think I [have decided] just to face reality. This is going on and all I can do is to be strong and face it."[96]

Narciso claimed that the legal fees had left her "financially crippled." By February 1977, legal costs incurred amounted to close to $50,000 for each of the women. As their defense attorneys expected the cost to eventually exceed many times that amount, they petitioned the court for attorney fees, expert fees, and related expenses. Narciso signed an affidavit of financial condition confirming her unemployment, absence of income, and expenditure of all her personal savings for payment toward legal costs already incurred in her defense. According to the affidavit, she retained the law firm "intending in good faith to rely on financial support to be raised on her behalf by her friends and supporters here and in the Philippines."[97]

Shortly after the FBI targeted Narciso and Perez for the VA murders and the two nurses sought legal representation, two groups emerged to raise funds for their defense and to disseminate information about the case: the Narciso-Perez Legal Defense Fund established in Michigan and the Chicago Support Group for the Defense of the Narciso-Perez Case. These groups targeted and attracted different communities in the Philippines and the United States. Cochaired by two doctors, Dr. Benes and Dr. Taylor, the Narciso-Perez Legal Defense Fund received financial support from professional organizations such as the Philippine Nurses Association and its overseas chapters in the United States and branches of the Philippine government such as the Philippine consulates. For example, during his visit to the Philippines, Dr. Benes received a donation of 5,000 pesos from the Armed Forces of the Philippines.

The leadership of the Chicago Support Group emerged from the KDP (Katipunan ng mga Demokratikong Pilipino), a primarily Filipino anti-imperialist and antiracist organization.[98] However, the group chose the name Chicago Support Group to distinguish itself from the KDP and to include other members of the Filipino community who did not necessarily espouse the political ideology of that organization. Although Chicago Support Group coordinator Esther Simpson was a member of the KDP and other members of the KDP were greatly involved in the Support Group effort, according to Simpson, "There were other members in the Filipino community who were not political at all, just plain members of the community, who were interested in this support for the nurses."[99]

While the Chicago Support Group, like the Narciso-Perez Defense Fund, participated in the effort to raise funds, it had a unique educational agenda. According to Simpson, aside from freeing the two nurses, vindicating them of the charges, and raising money for their defense, another main goal of the Chicago Support Group was "to educate the Philippine community particularly, and the American community, about racial and national discrimination," a major objective of the KDP. According to Simpson, the Narciso-Perez case was "a good case" for the KDP because, "first of all, these two women were nurses and in that area of the United States, in the Midwest, nurses form the bulk of the Filipino community. And it was very blatantly a case of racial and national discrimination brought about by the facts of how the two nurses were blamed for the murders." Although Simpson characterized discrimination as a "general Filipino experience" in the United States, it was an experience that was not often directly acknowledged nor understood: "[Filipinos in the United States] may have experienced discrimination, but they can't understand why they have to work as draftsmen when they were engineers in the Philippines. Why are they working as dental hygienists when they were all dentists in the Philippines?"[100]

Simpson observed that Filipinos in the United States questioned the case against Narciso and Perez given this "general experience" of discrimination. She continued, "Even though that is not spelled [out] clearly that that is discrimination, there is a gut feeling because of that general experience. That, oh, they chose them because they were Filipinos." Simpson also acknowledged the role that Filipinos' own essentialist beliefs about professional Filipino women played in their support for Narciso and Perez: "Filipinos have their own image that we can never do wrong. We are good people. And we can't believe they can do that. They are good nurses. They are graduates of good nursing schools."[101]

My interviews with Filipino nurses in the United States affirmed Simpson's observations. Several nurses acknowledged the role that discrimination had played in the case, but they did so in ambiguous, general ways, which questioned why Filipinos had been targeted for the crimes. For example, Milagros Rabara commented, "I thought they were not guilty . . . because there were other nurses on the floor and I don't know why these two were singled out." Similarly, Priscilla Santayana mused, "They were exploited and discriminated [against]. . . . And why were the two Filipinos singled out?"[102]

Many of the Filipino nurses referred to their strong belief in the essential goodness of Filipinos in general, and Filipino nurses specifically. Milavic Carroll claimed that she believed Narciso and Perez were innocent because "it's innate in Filipino nurses in general. They have compassion, devotion to be nurses. I don't think they're murderers." And Rosario DeGracia insisted, "We know they were innocent. It's unlikely that a woman and a nurse for that mater and Filipino in addition would commit such an atrocity." Corazon Guillermo pointed to Narciso's professional nursing training in the Philippines and concluded, "Narciso is from PGH [Philippine General Hospital]. They did not do it. How could someone with a sensible mind do this?" And Hermila Rabe stated, "I just feel strongly they are innocent because I don't think Filipinos will just poison those patients."[103]

Although Filipinos felt strongly about the innocence of Narciso and Perez, Esther Simpson believed that education about discrimination, specifically the ways the FBI and U.S. attorneys had scapegoated these Filipino immigrant women, was necessary to motivate people to organize and to donate funds. Her own commitment to defend the two nurses derived from her knowledge about broader issues of racism and discrimination that she had learned about when she became involved in antimartial law work. As she came to know antimartial law supporters from a community including but not limited to Filipinos, she related that she had been exposed to different literatures, "books that you never heard of before." Although Simpson herself is a Filipino nurse, she explained:

I did not know these two nurses at all. But I think it was really more the issue. Because during that time, it was not a complete experience of mine, but . . . the history of Filipinos in the U.S. had been around discrimination. If you look at different books, *America Is in the Heart* by [Carlos] Bulosan, and some experiences that may have followed afterward, like this accountant from California. She was a CPA in the Philippines, and was afterwards not allowed to be a CPA here. Around that time there were a lot of nurses who were being deported under the working visa. Why are we being treated so differently coming here as professionals, when in fact we don't have to be because we are professionals when we come over here? . . . After reading these books . . . if you study the history of how Filipinos were treated, how immigrants and minorities were treated, all the laws that came about, [for example] that Filipinos cannot marry white women. This is interesting.[104]

To accomplish the educational component of the group, Chicago Support Group members distributed educational brochures. They conducted door-to-door leafleting in apartment buildings where many Filipinos lived. For the majority of members, organizing around an issue like the Narciso-Perez case was a new experience. Some claimed that it was a rewarding experience because Filipinos were receptive to donating to the cause. Others learned about some of the issues that had inspired people like Esther Simpson to become activists. As one member observed as they conducted the door-to-door leafleting, "[Filipinos] usually end up sharing their experiences on how they are discriminated upon in their jobs."[105]

The Chicago Support Group attempted to involve as many Filipinos as possible in the effort by targeting spaces frequented by Filipinos. Aside from apartment buildings where many Filipinos lived, they leafleted, sold raffle tickets, and collected donations at work among Filipino colleagues, in stores with Filipino customers, and even at airports with *Balikbayan* travelers.[106] They transformed social events into fund-raisers; for example, a birthday party became a fund-raising event when guests gave donations to the defense fund instead of gifts.

Shortly after its formation, the Chicago Support Group decided to expand to other cities where there were subchapters of the KDP in place. According to Simpson, "A lot of Filipinos, when they heard about the case, there was a lot of sentiment of support for them. The thing was, how to channel this sentiment to the benefit of these nurses. And it really takes an organization to do that."[107] The KDP official newspaper and informational pamphlets publicized the need for support groups in other areas. Simpson related that she would offer guidelines and share experiences about how the Chicago Support Group had been established with the person from another area who was most interested in the case. As the group became national in scope, Jun Narciso, brother of Filipina, coordinated the local defense efforts in Chicago and Simpson became its national coordinator. By the time of the trial, Narciso-Perez support groups had formed in New York, Philadelphia, Washington, D.C., Boston, Atlanta, Cincinnati, Ann Arbor, Detroit, Sacramento, Oakland, San Francisco, Los Angeles, and San Diego; in Maryland, Connecticut, Maine, Indiana, Missouri, Texas, Hawai'i, and Guam; and in Vancouver, Toronto, and Montreal.

Although organizations with different political ideologies supported Narciso and Perez, they initially worked together in specific ways to increase the support for the two nurses. Simpson described these relationships as "polite." For example, the Chicago Support Group sold the Narciso-Perez Legal Defense Fund's raffle tickets. And the Defense Fund sold the Chicago group's "Free Narciso and Perez" T-shirts. However, Simpson believed that the membership of the Chicago Support Group distinguished it from the Narciso-Perez Legal Defense Fund. She characterized the Chicago group as a "grassroots" organization, in contrast to the Defense Fund, which for the most part was led by Philippine consulate groups, professional organizations, and social organizations. Filipino professional nursing organizations used their chapters as a springboard to organize and to collect money for the defense. The Philippine Nurses Association raised 650,000 pesos or $85,000 for the defense fund through its national network of PNA chapters. Filipino and Asian professional nursing organizations in the United States also responded to the need of Narciso-Perez defense committees. Members of the Filipino Nurses Association of Seattle and the Asian Nurses Association formed the Seattle Narciso/Perez Defense Committee. One of the main goals of a new PNA chapter in Ohio was to raise money for the defense. Simpson acknowledged the significance of the role these organizations played in galvanizing support for the two nurses. Although many of their supporters refused to picket or to wear the Support Group's T-shirts, Simpson admitted, "Filipinos belong to different organizations. Their annual dinner dances give them something to work on during the year. What keeps them together could just be social or regional. But it still serves a purpose."[108]

However, these "polite" relationships among various Filipino organizations in support of Narciso and Perez were fragile from the beginning. According to Simpson, pro-Marcos Filipinos attempted to discredit the work of the Chicago Support Group by labeling its members communists, even though some members had not been involved in any kind of leftist political activity. Simpson related that Chicago Support Group members then responded this way: "If we are communists, so be it. It doesn't take a communist to defend Narciso and Perez. We want them free."[109]

However, by the end of the trial in July 1977, the guilty verdict set in motion a series of hostile exchanges among various Filipino organizations that were publicized in the Filipino American press. Disagreement over their analyses of the guilty verdict and their strategies for challenging the verdict shattered the fragile alliance. In a *Filipino Reporter* article, several Filipinos (including leaders from the PNA and the Philippine Medical Association) argued that the guilty verdict was the result of the incompetence of Narciso and Perez's defense lawyers. They suggested that the nurses would not have been convicted had a Filipino lawyer from the Marcos government defended them, and subsequently recommended that future donations to the defense fund be withheld until both women changed their attorneys.

Both the Chicago Support Group and the KDP National Executive Board published editorials in response to these charges in the KDP newspaper, *Ang Katipunan*. In these editorials, the Chicago Support Group and the KDP defended the defense team against allegations of incompetence and praised their efforts to expose the weaknesses, irregularities, and discrepancies of the government's case. The Chicago Support Group characterized such allegations as a diversion from the main issue in the case, which they believed to be class-based, racial, and national discrimination. They claimed, "Leonora Perez and Filipina Narciso were convicted by the American judicial system which implements a lenient and flexible standard for the wealthy and powerful, and a harsh standard for the working people and the poor, where elements of skin color and national origin arbitrarily decide the judgment of the courts and legal apparatus."[110]

The KDP National Executive Board interpreted the charges as "a conscious attempt on the part of the Philippine consulates to sabotage the support movement." They believed that pro-Marcos Philippine consulate officials wanted to discredit the support movement because anti-Marcos groups, such as the KDP, were involved in organizing support for Narciso and Perez. The Board reiterated the Chicago Support Group's position that the main issue of the case was "racist, anti–foreign born prejudice" and then connected it with the repression of human rights by the Marcos government in the Philippines: "For the Marcos regime — which consistently represses the democratic rights of its own people — to be so concerned with the movement for democratic rights of minorities is just blatant hypocrisy. Marcos obviously prefers to have the Narciso/Perez conviction summarized as some freak miscarriage of justice due to 'incompetent' defense lawyers, rather than a frame-up of discrimination against minorities." Declaring an end to a coalition with such pro-Marcos supporters, the Board concluded, "This is the kind of 'support' the two nurses and the entire defense movement can do without."[111]

DOING WITHOUT, MOVING ON

Despite the split between pro- and anti-Marcos supporters, protests in support of Narciso and Perez intensified after the guilty verdict. Members of the Chicago Support Group held community meetings in a number of cities across the United States to discuss the verdict and to reorganize their protest efforts. Reflecting the Chicago Support Group's commitment to community organizing and grassroots support, these meetings in Chicago, New York, and San Francisco took place in Filipino community centers, such as the Jose Rizal Center in Chicago. They were also held in ecumenical centers, such as the United Nations Church Center in New York and Glide Church Freedom Hall in San Francisco.

According to Esther Simpson, over one hundred individuals and representatives from various Filipino organizations, the Black Panthers, Muslim national groups, and the U.S. Communist Party attended the Chicago and New York meetings. The Narciso-Perez case attracted the interest of diverse U.S. marginalized groups because Chicago Support Group members framed the case broadly as an issue of minority prejudice, with justice for all at stake. At the postconviction San Francisco community meeting, Vee Hernandez, member of the Bay Area Defense Committee for Narciso and Perez, claimed, "Now, with the conviction of Narciso and Perez, we have learned our bitter lesson — which is that American justice is a mockery." Hernandez connected the case against Narciso and Perez to "[the FBI's] history of repression particularly against minorities." And Jun Narciso reiterated, "This is not a fight for Leonie and [Filipina] alone but a fight for all minorities."[112]

While they emphasized political organizing and coalition building with other minority groups, Chicago Support Group members also articulated a collective Filipino American consciousness. A KDP member stated, "Whether this incident will go down in history as a testimony of our weaknesses as a minority or whether it will be remembered as a shining example of how we, as a minority, can unite and organize to correct an injustice — is also up to us." Margie Espina, president of the Philippine New York Jaycettes, insisted, "We have to organize! We have to join our little voices so that they may be heard. Alone I cannot do it! Alone you cannot do it! But all together, we have a better chance of accomplishing something! I have one question to ask: Shall we join together?"[113]

Supporters of Narciso and Perez demanded a new trial for the nurses through a nationwide publicity effort. They circulated a petition addressed to Judge Philip Pratt of Detroit to "Demand Justice . . . Free Narciso and Perez." The text of the petition claimed that Narciso and Perez were "targets of harassment" who had been "unjustly convicted," and criticized their trial as "marred" by the "withholding and tampering of evidence by the prosecution," "a long series of irregularities throughout the investigation," and "scanty 'evidence.'" Petitioners concluded, "We can only assume that Narciso and Perez have been convicted because of prejudice against their nationality."[114]

By November 2, the day that U.S. District Judge Pratt heard the arguments of the defense's motions for a new trial, approximately thirty-thousand petition signatures had been collected. Supporters rolled the petition sheets into large diploma-like rolls and presented them to court authorities in five boxes. Approximately two hundred supporters rallied outside the Detroit Federal Building, and similar rallies took place simultaneously in New York, Philadelphia, Seattle, Los Angeles, Sacramento, San Diego, San Francisco, Hawai'i, and Guam.

The Chicago Support Group also organized a national conference in

Chicago to strategize protest efforts after Judge Pratt's decision. Local support groups across the United States organized fund-raisers to defray travel costs for attending the conference. Like previous Narciso-Perez fund-raisers, these activities were social and community-based, featuring potlucks, skits such as "The VA Coverup," and disco dancing.

On December 19, 1977, Judge Pratt filed a fifty-eight-page opinion granting the defendants a new trial. Although Pratt had consistently denied the defense's motions for acquittal, his justification for a new trial reiterated the arguments that the defense attorneys had presented during the course of the original trial. Pratt criticized prosecution witnesses' eyewitness testimonies of the movements of the defendants, characterizing them as "confusing, inconsistent, and often hard to follow." He cast doubt on the choice of Narciso and Perez as number one suspects given that "security at the hospital was lax or almost non-existent." Pratt continued that "there was almost total freedom of movement for anyone dressed in conformance with the hospital custom." He acknowledged that the government failed to offer a motive to support its case against Narciso and Perez and that prosecution witnesses suffered from attacks on their credibility. He concluded, "The government's case was not strong and was entirely circumstantial."[115]

Chicago Support Group members celebrated the new trial, but also prepared to engage in more protest work. They continued to promote a Filipino American minority consciousness. One local support group, the Bay Area Defense Committee for Narciso and Perez, attempted to garner more support for the new trial by publicizing a history of discrimination faced by Filipinos in America:

> The Filipino community, in particular, has learned a very valuable lesson in the process of the defense movement: we must fight discrimination and stand up for our democratic rights. The discrimination so evident in this case has rudely reminded us that the history of the Filipino people in this country was always marked by racist and chauvinist attacks. In the '20s and '30s, discriminatory laws and practices were widespread. At its height, vigilante groups hunted down Filipinos in many parts of California and attacked them brutally. The worst attack was the "Watsonville Riot" when a meeting of Filipino farmworkers was shot at and a Filipino, Fermin Tobera, was killed. Today, Filipino immigrants continue to be hard hit by racism and national chauvinism and the Narciso and Perez case is symbolic of the many discriminatory incidents still experienced by Filipinos here in

the U.S. . . . Now that we have this new trial . . . we should not rest on our laurels. The fight is not yet over.[116]

The fight for Narciso and Perez's freedom continued until February 1978, when a new U.S. Attorney, James K. Robinson, filed a motion to dismiss the case against them. Robinson cited the lack of motive, circumstantial evidence, questionable eyewitness testimonies, and the absence of any previous criminal activity on the part of the defendants in his justification for dismissal. Although acknowledgment of these weaknesses of the government's case was hardly new, Robinson's other motivations for the dismissal revealed ironic reversals on the use of government resources and the significance of public opinion. At the beginning of the investigation, the government's seemingly unlimited resources and its desire to regain the public's confidence justified its aggressive investigation and development of the case against Narciso and Perez. However, by 1978 Robinson argued that concerns about government resources and public confidence merited dismissal. He claimed that a new trial would require substantial amounts of time and staff: "many months" and "the full time efforts of at least three Assistant United States Attorneys, not to mention the support services of law enforcement and clerical [personnel]." Robinson also pointed to the public's skepticism of the guilt of Narciso and Perez and, by extension, the American judicial system. He warned that "such expressions of public skepticism of the process by which persons are accorded due process in our criminal justice system are troublesome and bode ill for public confidence in our institutions."[117]

According to Esther Simpson, the dismissal of the remaining charges against Narciso and Perez was a Filipino "people's victory": "The most that I could appreciate from this work is that you could see how the Filipino community united around one issue that they believe in or they would want to work out. You could see the potential of the community, because if not for their efforts, P.I. and Leonie would just be anybody and they would be left on their own with a public defender, like most who don't have money. That was really great to see that the Filipino community worked around that."[118]

Although Filipinos continued to contact Chicago Support Group members such as Simpson about other discriminatory cases and issues, the group dissolved as an official group after U.S. Attorney Robinson dropped the case against the two nurses. Simpson recalled that a congressman from Los Angeles offered to sponsor a congressional hearing to work for another investigation of the VA deaths. However, Narciso and Perez did not want to participate in a new investigation. According to Simpson, she and other members of the Chicago Support Group keep in touch with Narciso and Perez, who live in Michigan and Southern California, respectively.

Filipino nurses across the United States had actively participated in the protests, but they had not done so in a singular or official organizational manner. Filipino nurse Simpson coordinated the national activities of the Chicago Support Group, but it was not a Filipino nurse organization. Other Filipino nurses in the United States, especially those in the Chicago and Detroit areas, protested the case in visibly significant numbers as they carried placards of support outside the courtroom. And still other Filipino nurses, such as those in Ohio and New Jersey, organized themselves into local PNA chapters to fund-raise more effectively and to educate themselves about their rights and responsibilities in the United States.

After the jury convicted Narciso and Perez in July 1977, Filipino nurses across the United States suffered from public suspicion about their professional intentions. One VA Hospital nurse in Philadelphia reported that she received a phone call from someone who threatened to kill the Filipino nurses of the hospital.[119] Filipino nurses across the United States reported instances of patients refusing to take medication from them and of hospitals developing policies not to hire Filipino nurses. The case against Narciso and Perez affected an entire group of foreign-trained nurses and led Filipino nurses to organize and participate in the protests, albeit in local and individual ways.

One of the impacts of the Narciso-Perez case was that it raised the consciousness of Filipino nurses in the United States, a consciousness of themselves as an immigrant, foreign-trained professional group in need of more complete awareness of their rights and obligations as foreign-trained nurses working in the United States. Although this new consciousness did not galvanize them to organize nationally as a professional group of Filipino nurses in the United States, by the late 1970s other nursing issues would.

CHAPTER 6

Conflict and Caring

Filipino Nurses Organize in the United States

In 1974, Elvie Santos (not her real name) faced deportation by the U.S. Immigration and Naturalization Service. She lamented, "I first came to the United States on Jan. 14, 1974 with the understanding that I would work as a nurse and make money — much more [than] what I was receiving as a nurse in the Philippines. I am so disappointed at the outcome or turn of events and now I am wondering if my coming here is worth my leaving my family behind."[1]

Originally, a U.S. recruitment agency had recruited Santos to work as a nurse in the United States after paying $100 to a Philippine agency. However, upon her arrival in Washington, the agency assigned her work as a nurses' aide in a nursing home. Elvie performed the duties of a registered nurse, but received half of an RN's salary. She then faced deportation proceedings in 1974 because she had worked in the United States under an H-1 or temporary work visa but had not passed the U.S. nursing licensure examination. Foreign-trained nurses were eligible for H-1 visa status only if they were licensed and employed as RNs in the United States.

In the mid-1970s, Filipino nurses entered the United States through new visa categories and encountered new licensing requirements. Philippine and U.S. recruitment agencies took advantage of these new migration opportunities by exploiting Filipino nurse migrants with misleading advertisements, low wages, and poor working conditions. By the late 1970s, exploitive recruitment practices, controversial licensing examinations, and a growing awareness of their complex and unique situation in the United States motivated Filipino nurses to organize. However, while many Filipino nurses in the United States were critical of these recruitment practices and licensing examinations, their critiques differed considerably. These differences led to the formation of three U.S.-national organizations: the National Federation of Philippine Nurses Associations in the United States (later renamed the National Organization of Philippine Nurses Associations in the United States and then the Philippine Nurses Association of America), the National Alliance for Fair Licensure of Foreign Nurse Graduates, and the Foreign Nurse Defense Fund.

This chapter analyzes the development of these organizations in the context of complex developments on both sides of the ocean during the 1970s. During this decade, the Marcos government's commitment to an export-oriented economy helped to transform Filipino nurses from national traitors into the Philippines' new national heroes. Although Philippine government officials appealed to Filipino nurses abroad to help a weak economy, Filipino nurses in the United States also felt a growing sense of alienation from Philippine nursing, in particular the Philippine Nurses Association. At the same time, however, xenophobic sentiments expressed by American nurses, including a commission of the American Nurses Association, transformed Filipino nurses from a welcome exchange visitor and immigrant into an alleged threat to the U.S. health care system.

The rhetoric of Philippine government officials and American nurses often rendered Filipino nurses as objects: objects of affection, objects of domestic production, and objects of international consumption. This chapter presents Filipino nurses as historical subjects who have struggled to ameliorate their situation as health professionals and Filipino Americans. By doing so, this history documents a rich diversity of Filipino nurse activism in the United States and challenges the prevailing view of Filipino women as docile and submissive.

However, this chapter also cautions against sweeping generalizations about Filipino nurses' political agendas. Although the xenophobic sentiments expressed by American nurses pitted American against Filipino nurses, divisions within the international nursing community could not be reduced to a simplistic dichotomy. Filipino nurses' creation of several U.S. national organizations illustrated that their agendas were distinct from those of nursing organizations in the Philippines. Furthermore, the presence of multiple Filipino nurses' organizations in the United States also reflected their diverse and competing interests within the United States. American nurses' opinions about new licensing examinations also diverged greatly. For example, individual American nurses opposed positions taken by the American Nurses Association, reflecting the inability of both U.S. and Filipino nursing organizations to unite nurses nationwide.

NEW CATEGORIES AND CONTROVERSIES

The controversy over U.S. nursing licensing examinations was linked to the creation of a new category of foreign nurse migrant, the H-I visa nurse. In the late 1960s and early 1970s, as the use of the Exchange Visitor Program decreased, occupational immigrant visas became the major avenue of entry for Filipino nurses wishing to work in the United States. However, as foreign professionals took advantage of available occupational immigrant visas, backlogs for these visas increased. By 1970, the waiting period for a third preference visa from the Eastern Hemisphere was approximately thirteen months.[2] In 1970, an immigration amendment dramatically increased employment opportunities for temporary foreign workers with H-I visas by allowing them to fill permanent positions.[3] The waiting time for an H-I visa was comparatively short; according to one placement agency, a qualified nurse's waiting period for an H-I visa was approximately thirty to ninety days.[4]

Nurses from the Philippines dominated the number of H-I visa nurses entering the United States. Between 1972 and 1978, 15,291 H-I visa nurses entered the United States; H-I visa nurses from the Philippines made up approximately 60 percent (9,158) of this total.[5] Canada was the second largest sending country of H-I visa nurses, with 3,034.[6]

Changes in the U.S. licensure of foreign-trained nurses placed H-I visa nurses at the center of a U.S. nursing controversy. In the United States, licensure for nurses is regulated by separate laws in each of the states. Before 1970, some states offered licensure to foreign-trained nurses by endorsement. For example, in the 1950s and 1960s in New York State, foreign-trained nurses individually petitioned the State Board of Regents for endorsement of their license and the board then evaluated each applicant. Reciprocity was often granted to Filipino nurses who had a license to practice as an RN in the Philippines.[7] Furthermore, given the increasing demand for nursing services, individual states implemented policies to ease the licensure process for foreign-trained nurses. In the 1960s, the temporary work permit for foreign nurses in New York was extended from six to eighteen months to give those foreign-trained nurses who did not have all the educational requirements for endorsement enough time to complete the necessary coursework.[8]

However, in 1971, New York State amended this approach. Foreign nurses were required to pass the State Board Test Pool Examination (SBTPE), an examination to test knowledge of U.S. nursing practice.[9] Five test areas — medical, surgical, psychiatric, obstetric nursing and nursing of children — composed the SBTPE. The National Council of State Boards of Nursing, a part of the American Nurses Association until 1978, developed the examination. Individual state licensing agencies then contracted with the National Council for its use. According to a 1975 report on foreign nurse graduates in the United States, the increasing cultural diversity, as well as numbers, of foreign nurses made individual evaluations more burdensome and problematic.[10] By 1977, all state boards abandoned licensure by endorsement and required foreign-trained nurses to take the SBTPE.

Some states, like Michigan, implemented policies that shortened the amount of time H-1 visa nurses could prepare for the examination. Before 1974, H-1 visa nurses in Michigan were issued a temporary work permit for six months after passing an English test; this permit was renewable for another six months. In 1974, a new regulation discontinued the renewal policy and compelled H-1 visa nurses to pass the SBTPE within six months.

The majority of foreign-trained nurses who took the SBTPE failed. According to a 1976 national report, the failure rate was 77 percent.[11] In individual states, rates were even higher. In New York, the failure rates of foreign-trained nurses taking the examination from 1972 to 1974 for the first time ranged from 63.6 percent to 90.9 percent. The failure rates of repeat candidates were also high, ranging from 52.2 percent to 86.6 percent.[12] In California, affirmative action officer Delfi Mandragon Shakra observed that 80 to 90 percent of Filipino nurses failed the examination in the 1970s.[13] These failure rates were particularly alarming when contrasted with those of U.S.-trained nurses, the vast majority of whom passed the SBTPE, at rates of 85 to 90 percent.[14]

Failing the examination was a potentially devastating experience. Weveline Aragon arrived in California in the late 1960s after four years of university training in nursing in the Philippines. She worked in Vallejo's Kaiser Hospital as a nurses' aide and, in 1971, enrolled in California State University at Chico to further her nursing training. Her fieldwork included leadership training at Providence Hospital, psychiatric nursing at CSU at Napa, and obstetric nursing at Travis Hospital. After graduating from CSU at Chico in 1973, Aragon took the SBTPE and failed. She then worked for the American Red Cross in Berkeley in safety and social services, took the SBTPE again, and failed again. She then applied for a position as the director of Nursing Services for the Oakland branch of the Red Cross with forty other applicants, and placed first. After working in this position for over a year, Aragon was given another chance to take the SBTPE, but was also warned of termination because she was not yet an RN. Aragon initially lamented, "I thought it was only me." However, she met many Filipino nurses at the state board examinations and observed that "the same people were turning up over and over again." Aragon circulated questionnaires among two hundred of them and found that since 1975, only one had passed the test. She reported that some had become so dehumanized over their repeated failures that they threatened suicide.[15]

Rosario DeGracia, a professor of nursing at Seattle University and president of the local Filipino Nurses Association, suggested that several factors contributed to these high failure rates. Filipino nurses' comparatively limited training in psychiatric nursing in the Philippines resulted in difficulty passing that area of the SBTPE. Some Filipino nurses also claimed that the multiple-choice format of the examination was confusing. In addition to these factors, DeGracia pointed out that "taking an examination can be a literally 'frightening' and anxiety-filled experience to those who have been away from school for many years."[16]

Failure of the examination had a detrimental effect on the visa status of H-1 visa nurses. Their temporary work visa status was revoked because, upon failing the licensing examination, they were unable to practice as registered nurses. Like Elvie Santos, they then faced the threat of deportation. These deportations profoundly affected individual hospitals that relied on the labor of H-1 visa nurses. For example, in 1975, immigration officers ordered thirty-five Filipino nurses to leave Pontiac, Michigan, after they failed the SBTPE and their temporary work permits had expired.[17] In Texas, one of the six states that employs the vast majority of foreign-trained nurses, the potential loss of this critical labor supply led to a battle between U.S. nursing and hospital professional associations over issues of authority and standards.

In Texas, the state hospital association's use of H-1 visa nurses incited a struggle over which group had the authority to decide who was qualified to practice professional nursing. The Texas Nurses Association argued that only the State Board of Nurse Examiners had that authority. The

Texas Hospital Association claimed that hospital physicians shared that authority.

The controversy was partly rooted in state nurse practice amendments that had passed in the late 1960s. In 1969, the Texas Nurses Association amended the state nurse practice statute to limit the practice of nursing to those who had passed the SBTPE. However, before the amendment was passed, the Texas Hospital Association and the Texas Medical Association managed to create an exclusion clause that allowed anyone working "under the control or supervision or at the instruction of" a physician to bypass the amendment.

The significance of these state nurse practice amendments became apparent in the early 1970s. During this period, the Board of Nurse Examiners in Texas granted temporary work permits to H-1 visa nurses until they passed the SBTPE. As these permits became available, the number of foreign-trained nurses working in Texas increased exponentially, from 60 in 1970 to 1,752 in 1973. However, their high failure rates on the SBTPE became a cause for alarm. Only one of every four or five foreign-trained nurses passed the examination. In 1973, the State Board of Nurse Examiners refused to grant temporary permits. As a result, the INS decided to stop issuing H-1 visas for Texas-bound foreign-trained nurses and informed H-1 visa nurses already in the state that their visas would be revoked if they did not pass the SBTPE. However, the Texas Hospital Association protested the decision, claiming that the removal of H-1 visa nurses from the Texas hospital workforce would be "a catastrophic experience for Texas hospitals."[18] It referred to the passage of its exclusion clause, which stated that anyone could practice nursing in a Texas hospital under the direction of a physician. The hospital association's lawyers successfully persuaded the INS to reverse its previous decision.

In a 1974 issue of *RN*, Rhea Felknor's special report "Trouble in Texas" presented H-1 visa nurses as a commodity, a "million-dollar investment" by Texas hospital administrators who had organized costly recruitment programs in England, Ireland, Scotland, South Africa, and the Philippines. Ruth Board, executive director of the Texas Nurses Association, criticized the INS decision as detrimental to American public safety: "The law is intended to protect the public, not the nurse. There is no measure in Texas other than the State Board Test Pool exams to assure the public that a nurse has the minimum competency necessary to provide safe nursing care."[19]

In the early 1970s, the struggle for control over nursing took place in specific states such as Texas. However, by 1974, the American Nurses Association had also become involved in the controversy over foreign-trained nurses, licensure, and practice, illustrating that this struggle had become national in scope.

PROFESSIONAL RESOLUTIONS AND PRESCREENING EXAMINATIONS

In June 1974, the American Nurses Association Commission on Nursing Services presented a resolution at the ANA biennial convention. Its objectives were twofold: to remove the preferential status of foreign nurses in U.S. immigration policies, and to support the authority of state nurses associations to evaluate the practice of foreign-trained nurses. However, whereas the Texas controversy focused on Texas hospitals' use of H-1 visa nurses who had high failure rates on the SBTPE, the ANA Commission's resolution lumped all foreign-trained nurses together. Of the resolution's twelve points justifying its objectives, three focused on the professional incompetence of foreign-trained nurses in general. The ANA Commission claimed that "many foreign graduates are *not prepared to work* in roles expected of them," "some employers place foreign nurse graduates in roles for which they are *unprepared,*" and "United States professional schools of nursing cannot provide sufficient educational programs to foreign nurses with *academic deficiencies.*"[20]

The resolution pitted the interests of U.S. nurses against those of foreign-trained nurses. The twelfth point insisted that U.S. citizens should be given priority in U.S. nursing education, suggesting that the educational needs of foreign nurses with "academic deficiencies" competed with those of American nursing students. Two other points characterized the presence of foreign-trained nurses in the United States as detrimental because they accepted "salaries lower than the acceptable rates for U.S. nurses" and they were "attracted to areas where U.S. nurses cannot find employment."

Clarita Miraflor, president of the PNA of Chicago, characterized the resolution as nativist and racist: "The implicit racism and know-nothing attitude that permeates this resolution has no place in our profession, which prides itself upon its dedication to the service of mankind."[21]

Miraflor and several other nurses, including Anne Zimmerman (executive director of the Illinois Nurses Association) and Ann Zercher (treasurer of the ANA), formed an ad hoc committee and worked on an alternative resolution regarding foreign nurse graduates. The participation of Zimmerman and Zercher revealed that although the ANA Commission's resolution pitted foreign nurses against U.S. nurses, not all U.S. nurses (and not even all ANA leaders) agreed with the ANA Commission's position.

Their alternative resolution downplayed a foreign-versus-U.S. dichotomy and instead emphasized the international mobility of all nurses by opening with the point that "the world-wide mobility of nurses is impeded by language difficulties and dissimilarities in educational preparation."[22] It highlighted the role that U.S. hospital recruiters played in the problems of foreign-trained nurses in the United States, and pointed out that some recruited nurses were uninformed about U.S. licensing requirements. It called for the ANA to collaborate with the International Labor Organization and World Health Organization in the elimination of misleading U.S. recruitment practices.

The ad hoc committee also proposed the creation of a prescreening examination for foreign-trained nurses. According to their resolution, "many problems could be eliminated if nurses had the opportunity to be tested for communication skills and professional preparation in their country of origin before migration."[23] The committee urged the ANA and other relevant U.S. national organizations to create this examination. The ANA hearing committee and house of delegates passed the alternative resolution with minimal opposition.

The adopted resolution's call for the creation of a prescreening examination for foreign-trained nurses was followed by a June 1975 conference in Maryland on foreign nurse graduates in the United States. Conference participants recommended the creation of an independent organization that would be in charge of the prescreening examination. In 1977, the ANA and the National League of Nursing cosponsored the creation of a new non-profit U.S. nursing organization, the Commission on Graduates of Foreign Nursing Schools (CGFNS). The Commission would oversee the implementation and administration of the prescreening examination, known as the CGFNS examination.

The CGFNS examination had two parts: a nursing competency section that included the five areas of nursing covered by the SBTPE and an

English-language competency section. The CGFNS contracted with the National League of Nursing to develop the nursing competency section at a cost of $120,640, and with the Educational Testing Service to develop the English competency section at a cost of $53,942. It administered the first CGFNS examination in thirty-two cities (including Manila) around the world on October 4, 1978.

The CGFNS leadership attempted to bridge the multiple concerns about foreign-trained nurses by emphasizing both American patients' safety and foreign-trained nurses' welfare. Executive Director Adele Herwitz acknowledged the "great disappointment" of foreign-trained nurses who failed their state board examinations: "They have often felt discriminated against and disenchanted with the United States. . . . [Others] have been hired as nurses' aides and then pushed into taking registered nurse responsibilities on unpopular night shifts and/or in out-of-the-way communities. This has not contributed to safe patient care."[24] Jessie Scott, president of the CGFNS Board of Trustees, reiterated these dual concerns: "The CGFNS examination . . . helps *protect those foreign nurses* who are not prepared for professional practice in this country against relocation costs, personal disappointment, and possible exploitation, and at the same time, it helps *assure the American health care consumer of minimum safe practices.*"[25]

However, the Commission, the INS, and the U.S. Department of Labor also used the CGFNS examination in ways that angered both American and Filipino nurses. In the October 1978 issue of the *American Journal of Nursing,* American nurses Bonnie Vowell and Mary Pat Colon wrote angry letters to the editor in response to the news about the development of a prescreening examination for foreign-trained nurses. They strongly criticized the cost of the development of the CGFNS examination, in particular a $346,173 grant from the Division of Nursing of the Department of Health, Education, and Welfare. In their letters, they echoed some of the sentiments of the ANA Commission on Nursing Services by characterizing all foreign-trained nurses as a dangerous import commodity and by presenting the interests of foreign nurses and U.S. nurses as mutually exclusive. Vowell wrote angrily, "The idea of pretesting is a good one, but please tell me why our tax dollars and professional organizations are paying for this, an import commodity, that is detrimental to the nursing profession in the U.S. . . . I do resent [the

$346,173 grant from HEW]. However, I really take issue with the use of ANA and NLN membership fees to help import nursing competition."[26]

The viewpoints of Vowell and Colon emphasized a "foreign versus U.S." nurse dichotomy and excluded the ways some foreign-trained nurses, such as Clarita Miraflor, had actively participated in U.S. professional nursing organizations. Vowell continued, "Nurses in this country are fighting for a new image, for better salaries, and for other things, and here is the ANA, our representative, helping undermine our efforts. These foreign nurses are not members of our professional organization. They do nothing to further our professional cause!"[27] Colon interpreted the use of funds for a prescreening examination as detrimental to American nursing students: "What is there to be gained by promoting immigration of foreign trained nurses while many young men and women here are unable to enter the profession due to lack of space in available schools? . . . Scholarships and traineeships for our own students are always in a precarious state. . . . Yet there are these thousands of dollars to spend on helping foreign-trained nurses immigrate."[28] These letters illustrate the way some American nurses conceptualized nursing as a nation-bound, as opposed to an international, profession.

While individual American nurses interpreted the CGFNS as beneficial to foreign-trained nurses and detrimental to U.S. nurses, some Filipino nurses took the opposite point of view, characterizing the Commission and its use of the CGFNS examination as "anti-Filipino." In 1979, the Commission's Executive Director Herwitz claimed that "the constant and on-going harassment from the various organized groups of Filipinos in this country" was a "major problem." Herwitz listed these groups' efforts to protest CGFNS policies at local, national, and international levels, which included "trying to have the state of Pennsylvania rescind the CGFNS non-profit status; charging the U.S. Postal Service to investigate CGFNS for using mail to defraud; distributing hostile and inaccurate news releases to all the media charging ANA, NLN, HEW, the Department of Labor, etc. with all kinds of discriminatory practices; trying unsuccessfully to get a national television network to 'expose' CGFNS; trying to ascertain the location of the five exam sites in the U.S. in order to disrupt the October exam conducted at these centers; trying to work through the United Nations to request the World Health Organization to bring CGFNS to the World Court on charges of discrimination."[29]

Although Herwitz acknowledged that multiple Filipino nursing organizations in the United States participated in these protest efforts, she lumped them together as Filipino perpetrators of CGFNS harassment. However, Filipino nurses' dissatisfactions led to the formation of three U.S. national organizations: the National Federation of Philippine Nurses Associations in the United States, the National Alliance for Fair Licensure of Foreign Nurse Graduates (NAFL-FNG), and the Foreign Nurse Defense Fund. Although these organizations claimed that they represented the interests of Filipino nurses in the United States, they had distinct agendas and interpretations of the 1970s controversy regarding licensure and foreign-trained nurses. National Federation leadership struggled for mainstream recognition of the contributions of Filipino nurses in the United States; NAFL-FNG leadership demanded an end to what they considered to be a culturally biased nursing licensure examination; and the Foreign Nurse Defense Fund utilized civil rights legislation to oppose what they considered to be a racist nursing licensure examination.

FROM OVERSEAS CHAPTERS TO NATIONAL FEDERATION

In 1979, members of local PNA chapters throughout the United States formed a new U.S. national nursing organization, the National Federation of Philippine Nurses Associations in the United States. While H-1 visa nurses' problems and the CGFNS controversy were the immediate concerns that motivated the formation of a U.S. national organization, its formation was also linked to the transnational origins of these local chapters and the changing relationship between them and the PNA in the Philippines.

In the 1960s and 1970s, Filipino exchange visitor and immigrant nurses in New York, California, Illinois, and Hawai'i established PNA organizations and then actively pursued affiliation with the PNA in the Philippines as overseas chapters. After receiving official recognition as an overseas chapter, PNA-Chicago leaders told the association in the Philippines that the "success of the organization lies in your hands. We are therefore hoping for your guidance and inspiration in all the things we do."[30] By the mid-1970s, overseas PNA chapters had also formed in Michigan, Philadelphia, New Jersey, and Galveston. The president of PNA-Michigan characterized the recognition of her chapter by the association in the Philippines as an accomplishment. Among its major aims was the maintenance of ties to the "mother organization."[31]

Transnational ties between the "mother organization" and its overseas chapters were maintained by the visits of PNA presidents to overseas chapters in 1973 and 1976.[32] Filipino nurses in the United States continued to organize under the auspices of the PNA as late as 1977, when Alicia Anloague Tupaz wrote to the president, explaining, "I am one of the Filipino nurses residing here in Ohio and at present a supervisor in a county hospital. I wrote you with the purpose of asking permission from you to organize a chapter here in Cleveland and the suburbs."[33]

However, while the PNA was helping some new chapters in the United States organize in the 1970s, dissatisfaction developed among some of the older chapters. Some had discontinued their affiliation with the PNA. Col. Winnie Luzon, PNA president from 1970 to 1974, visited New York City in 1973 to meet with the PNA–New York Board of Directors and convince them to rejoin as an overseas chapter. Luzon also visited PNA–Southern California leadership to do the same. She reported that after three meetings with the board of directors of PNA–Southern California, she was successful in "getting them back as a Chapter of our Association."[34] However, she was unsuccessful with PNA–New York.

Generational differences and bureaucratic inefficiency resulted in alienation from the PNA. In 1965, the Filipino Nurses Association of Hawai'i discontinued their overseas chapter affiliation with the national organization. According to Ines Viernes Cayaban, a former Hawai'i chapter president, "many of the older, active member[s] of the FNA are retired, some of them have died. . . . Most of the young nurses there now are Hawaii-born. . . . Their failure to get news or information from the mother organization in the Philippines made them feel they did not belong."[35] The PNA seemingly ignored even the most devoted chapters abroad, such as the PNA-Michigan. The PNA-Michigan president wrote to the organization, "I have been anxiously waiting receipt of our membership cards for 1974 and it seemed Col. Luzon never got my letter and your response proved that it did reach the Manila office . . . though we never received the membership cards. . . . we would like to receive copies of the Phil. Journal of Nursing regularly . . . (I have not received a single copy!)."[36]

While some of its overseas chapters discontinued their affiliations, the PNA continued to struggle against internal dissension among its members in the Philippines. At the same time, the newly established martial law regime appealed to professional organizations in the Philippines, including the PNA, to unify their constituents in the effort to strengthen national unity.[37] However, PNA members criticized the organization's use of proxy voting in its elections and decision making, and suspected censorship of this controversy about the organization in its official publication, the *Philippine Journal of Nursing.*[38] In addition, the rise of other Philippine national nursing organizations challenged its ability to unify and represent all Filipino nurses.[39] Given these pressures, although the PNA recognized and sought to alleviate the hardships of Filipino nurses abroad, it did so somewhat ambivalently. In 1967, the association expressed interest in working with the Philippine Department of Labor on recruitment practices, but only in an advisory capacity.[40] It was not until 1977 that the organization officially collaborated with the Department of Labor regarding the problems faced by Filipino nurses abroad.[41] Furthermore, it had little power to effect the high failure rate of Filipino nurses taking U.S. licensing examinations. In 1975, PNA President Fe Valdez attempted to help these Filipino nurses abroad by writing to ANA President Rosamund Gabrielson, proposing that Filipino nurses be given three chances to pass the examination before their right to practice was fully revoked. In her response, Gabrielson implicitly rejected the proposal by simply pointing out that licensure for nurses in the United States was regulated by separate laws in each of the states.[42]

At first, PNA chapters in the United States attempted to alleviate problems regarding H-1 visa nurses and licensure on an individual chapter basis. For example, PNAs in Chicago, Washington, D.C., Southern California, Michigan, New Jersey, and New York offered licensing review courses and tutorials at minimal or no cost. The PNA-Michigan sponsored a roundtable with recruitment agencies to reduce placement fees and to improve orientations for newly arrived foreign nurses.[43] It also sent a delegation to meet with Governor Milliken to protest the deportations of the thirty-five Filipino nurses from Pontiac, Michigan.[44]

However, by 1979 PNA leaders in the United States recognized that these problems were similar in many states across the country. According to the minutes of the national organizational meeting, local PNA leaders concluded that, "after much deliberation and discussion, a decision was reached that we formally organize because of the pressing problem on [H-1] visa confronting the Filipino nurse and only through concerted effort of all PNAs we may be able to alleviate the problems affecting the Filipino nurses in the United States."[45]

PNA leaders in the United States also opposed the ways U.S. nursing organizations implemented the CGFNS examination. First, they opposed the mandatory use of CGFNS testing in the United States. The Commission had conducted research on foreign-trained nurses who had entered the United States as dependents of U.S. citizens and concluded that this group of foreign-trained nurses needed to pass the examination before taking the SBTPE. According to the CGFNS study, 0.7 percent of 4,500 women entering the United States as dependents were nurses. Despite this minuscule percentage, a Commission member concluded that "the Commission will have to consider how to handle this group, who will require pre-screen testing in this country."[46] As a result, the Commission offered the examination in Los Angeles, Chicago, and New York, claiming, "in this way, these nurses will not have to return to their country to take the CGFNS exam."[47] The PNA–New York met with the New York State Nursing Association's Human Rights Committee to protest CGFNS testing in the United States. They claimed that this rule appeared to contradict the Commission's purpose of screening foreign nurses "while they are still in their own countries." They questioned, "Why is the CGFNS examination imposed on these nurses that are already in the U.S. when the State Board examination alone is final in meeting the same purposes?"[48]

Second, PNA leaders in the United States criticized the use of the examination as a visa requirement. In 1977, the Commission convened a meeting with divisions of the INS, U.S. Department of State, and U.S. Department of Labor to lobby for the use of the CGFNS certificate in the visa applications of foreign nurse graduates.[49] Although only twenty-five state boards of nursing required the certificate from foreign nurse graduates before they could take the SBTPE in 1981, the Commission successfully persuaded U.S. government agencies to use the CGFNS certificate as a prerequisite for the issuance of immigrant and nonimmigrant visas to foreign nurses.[50] In January 1980, the INS declared that all professional nurses seeking permanent labor certification to immigrate to the United States would have to document a passing score on the CGFNS examination or the state licensing examination.[51] In April 1980, the INS further required that nonimmigrant nurses possess either the CGFNS certificate or a valid state license to practice nursing to qualify for an H-1 visa.[52] Because the SBTPE was not administered overseas, these new federal regulations compelled foreign nurses to pass both the CGFNS examination in the Philippines and the SBTPE in the United States.

Clarita Miraflor, who became the first president of the National Federation, claimed, "The concept of a visa qualifying exam is highly discriminatory." Objecting to its use on "humanitarian" grounds, Miraflor pointed to those Filipino nurses who had waited up to ten years for their H-1 visa and would have been denied a visa if they failed the CGFNS exam.[53] The use of the CGFNS certificate as a prerequisite for a visa significantly reduced the pool of Filipino nurses eligible to enter the United States. Although the Commission did not release country-specific pass and fail rates, the overall international pass rate after the first seven CGFNS qualifying examinations was 33 percent.[54]

Third, Filipino nurses criticized what they considered to be an exorbitant examination fee of $70, which in the Philippines during the late 1970s was equivalent to approximately one and a half months of a Filipino nurse's salary.[55] Maria Couper, PNA-Chicago president, characterized the Commission together with Philippine recruitment agencies and U.S. employers as exploiters of Filipino nurses.[56] According to Couper, as she urged other PNAs in the United States to adopt PNA-Chicago's critical position on the CGFNS examination, the need for a national organization became more apparent. Thus, the immediate concerns of H-1 visa nurses' problems and CGFNS policies combined with increasing dissatisfaction with the PNA in the Philippines to inspire representatives from New Jersey, New York, Chicago, Southern California, and Michigan to form the National Federation of Philippine Nurses Associations in the United States.

The National Federation acknowledged the uniqueness of its constituency through its ANA-influenced constitution and active communication with both U.S. and Philippine national nursing organizations. According to the chair of the by-laws committee, Filipinas Lowery, they had patterned the National Federation's by-laws after U.S. professional nursing organizations "because the people that we're serving are here [in the United States]."[57] However, the National Federation also continued to maintain dialogue with the PNA. For example, in June 1981, members of the National Federation (who officially renamed the organization the

National Organization of Philippine Nurses Associations in the United States or NOPNAUS that year) met with the PNA president to discuss problems regarding Filipino nurses' recruitment, licensure, and practice in the United States. As NOPNAUS attempted to unify Filipino nurses in the United States, their appeals to unity were challenged by the rise of other organizations.

FAIR LICENSURE: A CAUSE FOR THE FILIPINO COMMUNITY

During a two-day conference in 1977, over one hundred Filipino nurses and community activists formed the National Alliance for Fair Licensure of Foreign Nurse Graduates. The National Federation had attempted to unite Filipino nurses specifically; by contrast, the Alliance included Filipino nonnurses as well as nurses. Its national co-coordinators included community activist Aimee Cruz and registered nurse Christina Hing. Organized by the KDP, whose members had also organized the Chicago Support Group for the Defense of the Narciso-Pérez Case, the NAFL-FNG attempted to unify all Filipinos in the United States on the basis of their "minority" status.[58] The organization argued that the fair licensure of foreign-trained nurses was a problem for the entire Filipino community because "the nature of the problem clearly challenges our commitment and ability as a minority group to unite and fight discrimination in any area — whether in employment, housing, education, and others."[59]

The NAFL-FNG called for the simplification of English in the CGFNS examination, an investigation of cultural biases in the SBTPE, a minimum eighteen-month temporary license for foreign-trained nurses in the United States, and the establishment of licensure examination review programs in educational institutions throughout the United States. They advocated for "deferred voluntary departure" status, which would enable H-1 visa nurses who failed the SBTPE to obtain another opportunity for legal employment.

At the 1977 conference, Aimee Cruz urged participants to "depart from our traditional notion of conferences as 'talk festivals' where nice sounding resolutions are passed on paper and remain on paper."[60] That year, the NAFL-FNG launched a petition campaign addressed to INS Commissioner Leonel Castillo demanding deferred voluntary departure status for H-1 visa nurses who had failed the SBTPE. In 1978, it conducted another petition campaign addressed to Secretary Joseph Califano Jr. of the Department of Health, Education, and Welfare to demand low-cost and specialized review centers for foreign-trained nurses. In October 1979, the NAFL-FNG organized pickets in Los Angeles, Chicago, and New York to protest the use of CGFNS examinations in the United States.

The NAFL-FNG differed from the National Federation in its views on the U.S. nursing licensure examination. According to NAFL-FNG member Trinity Ordona, the test did not take into account language or cultural differences. She claimed, "The Alliance is calling for, first, the simplification of language in the tests. Secondly . . . there is the problem of an inadequate adjustment period. [Professional organizations] are blaming it on the Filipinos, but the bottom line is that they think foreign nurses are inferior."[61] However, some National Federation leaders disagreed with the claim that the licensure examination was biased. According to Filipinas Lowery, "For some reason there was this radical group of nonnurses going around saying that the licensing exam was discriminatory. And what we said was . . . being that we're nurses, we recognize that there's one exam to be taken by everybody. Whether you're American-educated or foreign-educated, you've got to meet one standard."[62]

However, a 1980 Adverse Impact Assessment report by the California Department of Consumer Affairs supported NAFL-FNG claims of cultural bias and further concluded that the SBTPE was racially biased. According to the report, 45 percent of Asians, 62 percent of Blacks, 55 percent of Filipinos, 40 percent of Latinos, and 40 percent of Native Americans failed the SBTPE, in contrast to the 12 percent failure rate of white test takers.[63] As a result, the NAFL-FNG participated in a coalition with organizations including the Service Employee International Union Locals 400 and 723, Asian Law Caucus, Mexican American Legal Defense and Education Fund, National Association for the Advancement of Colored People, Chinese for Affirmative Action, and the National Organization for Women, Bay Area, among others. This coalition supported a proposal to extend the temporary work permits of foreign-trained nurses to twenty-four months.[64] The NAFL-FNG also collaborated with immigrant advocacy organizations, such as the National Filipino Immigrant Rights Organization. Together they organized an emergency campaign demanding that the INS stop the deportations of H-I visa nurses until a "bias-free licensure exam" could be developed.[65]

DEFENDING FOREIGN NURSES: "COOLIES OF THE MEDICAL WORLD"

In the late 1970s, Filipino nurses organized yet another group, the Foreign Nurse Defense Fund, which defended the rights of foreign nurses in the United States through the use of civil rights legislation. Filipino nurse Norma Ruspian Watson was the executive secretary of the organization. Personal experiences of discrimination in the United States informed her activism. Watson arrived in the United States in 1973 with an occupational immigrant visa and passed the licensure examination in 1974. She and seven other Filipino nurses applied for employment at the Letterman Army Medical Center (LAMC). According to Watson, "we were all denied employment applications, and I was told to my face that LAMC does not hire brown skinned Fillippinas [*sic*]"[66] She later applied for work in a private hospital, Mary's Help Hospital in Daly City. In 1979, Watson filed a complaint with the Equal Employment Opportunity Commission after discovering that she was not being compensated for her seven years of professional nursing experience in the Philippines but was being paid as a new nursing graduate.[67]

Watson conducted research into the problems of other Filipino nurses in the United States. In her letter to President Ronald Reagan on behalf of the Foreign Nurse Defense Fund, she accused the National League of Nursing of violating state and federal civil rights through its development of a "racist and discriminatory" licensing examination. After securing documents through the Freedom of Information Act, she also accused government officials from the Department of Health, Education, and Welfare and the INS of "criminal conspiracy" through their use of the SBTPE as a basis for deportation of foreign nurses in the United States.[68] In a letter to the U.S. Commission on Civil Rights, Watson argued, "Foreign nurses, particularly Fillippinas [*sic*] are the "COOLIES OF THE MEDICAL WORLD," we have educated ourselves in our countries of origin at no cost to the American taxpayer, and all you have to do today, is look in any hospital in America and you will see our brown faces everywhere you look. We are sick and tired of being subservient and culturally non-aggressive, and now are taking pages out of the black Civil Rights Movement in this country, and will do what Martin Luther King had done. I would like to see all foreign nurses walk out of the hospitals in this country, and see what happens."[69]

Watson's vision of a foreign nurses' walkout never materialized. My research findings suggest that the NAFL-FNG and Foreign Nurse Defense Fund dissolved in the early 1980s. Political gains contributed to their demise. In 1981 in California the coalition of organizations successfully persuaded the state's Board of Registered Nursing to break away from the national nursing establishment by developing its own non-discriminatory and job-related licensure examination. The state board also decided to extend the temporary visas of thousands of foreign nurses who faced possible deportation after failing the controversial SBTPE. In July 1982, the National Council of State Boards of Nursing replaced the SBTPE with a new examination. The NCLEX-RN examination was designed in a way that permitted nurses to take the examination an unlimited number of times without compromising testing accuracy.

New political, labor, and personal conflicts also hastened the end of these organizations. Different revolutionary movements had divided KDP members (who had organized the NAFL-FNG) and led to the dissolution of the KDP in July 1986.[70] By the mid-1980s, Norma Watson had become embroiled in a hospital controversy about the use of protective clothing when taking care of AIDS patients. Watson filed a lawsuit after developing a virus common to AIDS patients she had treated at San Francisco General Hospital, claiming that the virus caused birth defects in her son.[71]

Only NOPNAUS remained active throughout the 1980s, a period marked by the political domination of Ronald Reagan and the Republican Party and rollbacks in race-, gender-, and class-based organizing. Its focus on mainstream recognition and integrationist tactics complemented this conservative political environment; it also reflected what Rick Bonus has found to be a pattern in Filipino American styles of politicking. According to Bonus, common concerns of Filipino American organizations include "their emphasis on recognition and group action. 'Doing politics' for them is always an effort, first, to calculate and respond to the effects, in the past and present, of having no representation in mainstream politics and no access to it, and second, to facilitate the establishment of self-reliant networks of support and mutuality—appropriated from the homeland—as alternative spaces of collective action."[72]

Thus, the recognition of the collective presence of Filipino nurses was a major concern for NOPNAUS leadership. When I asked Phoebe Cabotaje-Andes, who became the second president of NOPNAUS, from 1982 to 1984, if the ANA influenced its activities, she responded, "I don't think so. We wanted probably to be *recognized by the ANA* and that's why, when there was a convention in Louisiana, we participated by offering a program in their workshop." Cabotaje-Andes characterized NOPNAUS's presentation of the program "The Asian Nurse in the Health Care Delivery System: Issues and Trends in the 1980s" at the ANA's 1984 convention as one of the major achievements of her presidency. She related, "I thought that was giving us a positive image. It made us probably think we are a large, cohesive, and powerful group *in the eyes of the Americans,* being printed in the whole program . . . to get into the program was an accomplishment."[73] During Maria Couper's presidency from 1984 to 1986, she continued to pursue ANA recognition by successfully negotiating with the ANA to include NOPNAUS in the procession of dignitaries during ANA conventions' opening ceremonies.

Although NOPNAUS leadership attempted to present an image of their organization as "large," "cohesive," and "powerful," the organizational histories of the NAFL-FNG and Foreign Nurse Defense Fund challenge these images of unity and cohesion. Problems regarding foreign-trained nurses, licensure, and practice had divided Filipino nurses in the United States. As they protested exploitation, their conflicting agendas revealed the professional and political diversity among them and ultimately limited their ability to effect changes in U.S. nursing licensure and transnational recruitment practices. The controversial use of the CGFNS examination continued in most states through the 1990s, as did exploitive recruitment practices.

On December 18, 1989, Congress passed the Immigration Nursing Relief Act.[1] The Act enabled H-1 visa nurses who were present in the United States on September 1, 1989, and had worked for three years as a registered nurse in the United States, to adjust their status to permanent resident. It exempted H-1 visa nurses and their immediate family members from current immigrant visa numerical limitations and backlogs. Through their passage of this legislation, Congress members acknowledged the critical role that this group of nurses plays in the contemporary U.S. hospital workplace and other medical facilities.

However, the Immigration Nursing Relief Act also attempted to institutionalize the end of U.S. hospitals' recruitment of foreign-trained nurses. Congress members took seriously the concerns of American nurses who had argued that the presence of foreign-trained nurses in the United States adversely affected their employment opportunities. The second major feature of the 1989 Act was the establishment of a complex, multifaceted attestation requirement for those U.S. hospitals interested in hiring new nonimmigrant nurses. This feature required that these hospitals attest to a critical need for nonimmigrant nurses' labor, the absence of an adverse effect on the wages and working conditions of the hospitals' other registered nurses, the payment of the same wage rate for nonimmigrant RNs and other RNs similarly employed, and an active effort to recruit and retain American workers.

However, the U.S. government's ability to control future migrations of foreign-trained nurses to the United States and to ensure fair working conditions for both foreign-trained and American nurses was limited. In January 1998, Billy Denver Jewell, Holly Arthur Estreller, Sidney and Veronica Hewitt, and Haesook Kim pleaded guilty to illegally bringing hundreds of registered nurses from the Philippines into the United States to work in convalescent homes and other medical facilities. Expecting wages of $13 to $15 per hour, these nurses earned as little as $5 per hour as nursing assistants.[2]

Using the provisions of the 1989 Act, Jewell petitioned the INS and the Department of Labor for the use of Filipino nurses' labor in twenty-two nursing homes that he owned. However, the Hewitts and Kim recruited at least fifty of these nurses to work in medical care facilities throughout the country at substandard wages. They paid Jewell $1,000 to $1,500 for each illegal visa. This complex system was profitable for Kim and the Hewitts as well as Jewell because the recruited Filipino nurses paid up to $7,000 each to Kim and the Hewitts for these fraudulent visas. These actions illustrate the persistence of Filipino nurses' desire to work in the United States as well as the commodification of their labor; they also hint at some of the dynamics of Filipino nurse migration to the United States in the late twentieth century, such as the increasing desperation of Filipino nurses to work in the United States, the decrease in avenues for legal migration to the United States, and the emergence of new forms of profit making and exploitation by American recruiters.

Furthermore, despite the attempts to decrease the use of foreign nurses in the United States, the phenomenon of Filipino nurse migration has not abated. Today foreign nurses provide a critical source of labor for hospitals in the United Kingdom and Singapore, illustrating one way that the United States has become much more like (as opposed to exceptional or distinct from) other highly developed countries. Between 1998 and 1999, the number of foreign-trained nurses in the United Kingdom increased by 25 percent.[3] According to Singapore Minister of Health Yeo Chow Tong, without foreign nurses, "some of our services would be decimated."[4] U.K. as well as Singaporean recruiters targeted Filipino nurses because, according to some U.K. recruiters, "the Philippines seems a natural place to start — there is a culture of young people going abroad to work and the standard of English among potential recruits is excellent."[5]

Paul Ong and Tania Azores further observe that, even in the United States, "the pressure to recruit and admit more foreign nurses will continue. Although the latest immigration laws have placed new restrictions on the future importation of foreign nurses, historical evidence suggests that exceptions will once again be made as the needs arise."[6] A bill sponsored by U.S. representative Bobby L. Rush that would become the 1999 Nursing Relief for Disadvantaged Areas Act affirmed their prediction. The Act established a nonimmigrant visa for foreign RNs to work in areas hard-hit by staffing shortages. Rush sponsored the bill after critical nursing shortages almost caused St. Bernard Hospital in Chicago to close in 1992.[7] In the first few years of the new millennium, medical facilities in Wisconsin and Minnesota have aggressively recruited Filipino nurses to alleviate their local nursing shortages. In 2001, a group from the Wisconsin Association of Homes and Services for the Aging went to the Philippines and hired 70 nurses.[8] In 2002, a group of Filipino nurses arrived in the Twin Cities after several Twin Cities health-care organizations hired more than one hundred Filipino nurses as part of recruiting efforts that began in 1999.[9] Previously conceptualized as a primarily East and West Coast phenomenon, this aggressive recruitment of Filipino nurses to care for populations in the Midwest illustrates the way global and transnational forces continue to transform the "heartland of America."

Ong and Azores also surmise that Filipino nurses will continue to alleviate these U.S. nursing labor demands, given that "economic conditions in the Philippines are still precarious, and any improvement will not soon close the huge wage differences between the two countries."[10] In addition, the Philippine government continues to actively promote labor export abroad to accumulate much needed foreign currency as well as to alleviate Philippine unemployment. In a 1992 speech, Philippine President Fidel Ramos declared, "There are many countries in the world today which have adopted in one form or another a strategy of overseas employment, yet in no country has this program become so critical as it is for the Philippines today. . . . At some point, we've got to rein in the export of Filipino labor and turn it instead to development enterprises here at home. But until that time comes, when our country can fully absorb the energies of our labor force, overseas employment must remain an important part of public policy and a pillar of national life."[11] Given the country's massive $46 billion debt to the World Bank, International Monetary Fund, and other lending institutions based in North America, it seems unlikely that the export of Filipino laborers abroad will end or even decrease in the near future, when overseas workers' remittances have been the country's largest source of foreign exchange. According to the Central Bank of the Philippines, between 1975 and 1994 Filipino overseas contract workers sent remittances totaling $18.196 billion.[12]

Filipino women continue to play a significant role in this phenomenon. In 1991, they constituted a larger proportion of the Philippine's overseas workforce (41 percent) than its domestic workforce (36 percent), forming a worldwide diaspora of Filipino women working in Japan, Canada, the Middle East, several European countries, as well as the United States. Although the phenomenon of Filipino nurse migration abroad initiated the feminization of the contemporary Filipino overseas workforce, today the majority (approximately 70 percent) of Filipino women workers overseas are domestic workers. Significant numbers of Filipino women also work overseas in entertainment and sex industries.[13] While these different groups of overseas workers need to be studied on their own terms, the feminization, racialization, and commodification of these laborers as well as the degrading stereotypes that often accompany these processes bind them together in the new millennium. In 2001, Cheri A. Nievera, president of the Philippine Nurses Association of Greater St. Louis, wrote to the *St. Louis Post Dispatch* about an article the paper had recently published on newly recruited Filipino nurses at Barnes-Jewish Hospital. The article referred to the Filipinos as "mail-order nurses." Nievera critiqued this representation: "Last I checked, people who moved to the United States . . . were called immigrants, then citizens and, most importantly, members of a thriving, diverse community. Who knows? One day you may wake up to see a 'mail-order nurse' at your bedside taking excellent care of you. Filipino nurses are professionals, and we deserve respect, not belittlement."[14]

The presence of a Philippine Nurses Association in St. Louis further reminds us that recent legislative attempts to control the future migrations of foreign nurses into the United States cannot undo the incorporation of Filipino nurses already in these institutions. Four decades of active recruitment of Filipino nurses as exchange visitors, immigrants, and temporary workers have created a critical mass of these professional workers in hospitals and other medical institutions across the country.[15] In the late 1980s and 1990s, their presence continued to be at the center of controversies about U.S. culture and identity, such as the English-only movement.

In 1988, a new policy in the maternity ward of Pomona Valley Hospital Medical Center prohibited the Filipino nurses in the unit from speaking Tagalog at work under any circumstances, even during breaks and personal phone calls. Thus, although assistant head nurse Aida Dimaranan and two other Filipino nurses spoke Tagalog quietly to one another during a dinner break, according to Dimaranan, a supervisor who overheard them warned them "not to speak in [the] Filipino language because it was rude." Hospital supervisors claimed that the policy was enforced to improve working relations in the unit, relations they believed had been strained by Filipino nurses' use of Tagalog on the job. However, Dimaranan and other Filipino nurses at the hospital believed that the new policy only strained these relations further. Dimaranan claimed that the policy was "embarrassing and humiliating. We weren't doing it to deceive anyone. We are professionals." After Dimaranan challenged the no-Tagalog policy at hospital meetings, her previously positive work record suffered from poor performance evaluations, which resulted in a demotion. Like so many other Filipino nurses in the United States, she reflected romantically about her initial desire to come to America: "I always wanted . . . to come to America. To me it was such an exciting country." However, the hospital's implementation of a no-Tagalog policy and her subsequent demotion tempered her initial enthusiasm. Dimaranan lamented, "Twenty-five years of nursing, and it's crumbled."[16]

Dimaranan fought back, however, charging the hospital with work discrimination that violated Title VII of the Civil Rights Act of 1964. In 1991, the Central District Court of California awarded Dimaranan back pay and fringe benefits that she had been entitled to as an assistant head nurse from the time the case had been heard until the date of entry of the judgment. It also ordered her reinstatement to a job position equivalent to her previous position as assistant head nurse as well as the removal of the poor performance evaluations.[17] Although the court did not view the maternity unit's no-Tagalog rule as an English-only policy, the Tagalog controversy at Pomona Valley Hospital occurred only two years after the overwhelming passage of California's Proposition 63, which intended "to preserve, protect, and strengthen . . . English."[18] In 1994, the U.S. Supreme Court ruled that requiring bilingual workers to speak English on the job did not violate federal antidiscrimination laws. The *Los Angeles Times* interviewed Dimaranan about her reaction to the Supreme Court ruling. She responded that although she thought it was improper to speak a language other than English in front of a patient who speaks English only, she would not restrict nurses from speaking their first language in other situations. She explained, "Maybe I can express what I want to say in English. But it is just so different, better when I can say it in my own language. I'm not just speaking for my own feelings but for Vietnamese and Korean nurses. When I see them speaking their language, I feel better. I don't feel like it's rude."[19]

Dimaranan's desire to come to the "exciting country" of the United States and her struggles over language, professionalism, and performance in the U.S. hospital workplace speak to the importance of the cultural terrains that are often subsumed by an economic logic of wage differentials and workers' remittances, a logic that continues to dominate explanations of the contemporary phenomenon of Filipino nurse migration. The predominance of this economic logic contributes to the troubling commodification of Filipino nurse migrants as units of labor, which then potentially leads to insidious conclusions that Filipino nurse migrants financially benefit from and, thus, should be grateful for the opportunities they have to work abroad.

In this book, I have argued that this economic logic does not fully explain why Filipino women have become the quintessential foreign nursing care providers for highly developed countries such as the United States. I have emphasized the significance of the social and cultural as well as economic motivations of Filipino nurse migrants and other participants in this phenomenon (U.S. and Philippine governments, hospital recruiters, and professional nursing organizations) in shaping the transnational dynamics of this migrant flow over time. The 1999 comment by U.K. recruiters that "the Philippines seemed a *natural* place to start" for nurse recruitment suggests that Filipino women are inherently caring and nurturing and that the Philippines is somehow predisposed to the export of its young people. In doing so, it reflects the lack of historical understanding of this global phenomenon.

As I have argued, the development of this international professional labor force and the origins of Filipino nurse migration are not solely the results of contemporary global restructuring, but rather are historical outcomes of early twentieth-century U.S. colonialism in the Philippines. A culture of U.S. imperialism informed the creation of an Americanized training hospital system in the Philippines as well as new socioeconomic desires among Filipino nurses that would eventually prepare and motivate more of them to work abroad than in the Philippines. In the 1950s and 1960s, U.S. exchange programs and new occupational immigrant visas helped to transform previous colonial migrations of a Filipino nursing elite into mass migrations of Filipino nurses to the United States, migrations that refashioned, but ultimately perpetuated, racialized hierarchies. Despite the critical role that Filipino nurses have played in U.S. hospitals with nursing shortages, a culture of U.S. imperialism continued to inform the reception and incorporation of Filipino nurse migrants in the United States in the late twentieth century, stereotyping them as inferior and, at times, even dangerous. Filipino nurse activist

Norma Ruspian Watson pointed to the persistence of these imperial racialized and gendered hierarchies when she posed the question, "Do we bring our nursing skills to the USA as professionals, and to fill a needed medical health care crisis as such, or are we brought to the USA as their little brown-skinned sisters to empty bedpans and work in nursing homes?"[20] America's early twentieth-century empire in the Philippines inadvertently shaped these complex dynamics of this contemporary "empire of care."

A study that takes seriously the transnational dynamics of Filipino nurse migration requires a two-shores approach. My methodology included ethnographic and archival research in both the United States and the Philippines. As larger studies of migration often focus on the broader political and economic contexts in which migrations take place at the expense of the personal stories of migrants themselves, one of my objectives was to place a human face on this study through in-depth oral interviews with Filipino nurses in the United States. I conducted forty-three oral interviews, each lasting between one and three hours. Forty of these interviews were with Filipino nurses working in New York City hospitals (where the percentage of Filipino registered nurses is the highest in the United States) and took place in New York City. One interview took place in New Jersey; the remaining two were conducted in Washington State. Although the presence of Filipino nurses in nursing homes and other health care–related institutions has become more visible in recent years, the labor of Filipino nurses in U.S. hospitals is particularly significant. According to Paul Ong and Tania Azores, a 1984 study revealed that an overwhelming majority of Filipino registered nurses in the United States, over 82 percent, worked in hospitals, compared to 53 percent of non-Filipinos.

I recruited interview participants primarily using a snowball technique, in which I asked people for names of other potential participants. My Filipino immigrant family also got involved in this process by asking nurses they knew (or even had just met) if they might consider being interviewed by me. I am indebted to all of them, especially my mother, for her assistance in this regard because I believe that many of the nurses I interviewed saw me in the context of my family relations and that this context furthered their willingness to talk with me about their life history. My observations during two months of volunteer work at Bellevue Hospital in New York City and attendance at a Philippine Nurses Association of Southern California meeting in Fullerton and a Philippine Nurses Association of America conference at Las Vegas as well as my reading informed my interview questions.

In the United States, I conducted archival research at Boston University's nursing archives, the Filipino American National History Society archives in Seattle, Washington, and university libraries throughout the country to locate issues of the *Philippine Journal of Nursing,* mainstream and ethnic newspapers, American nursing journals and fact books, government documents, and federal court records. The voluminous records of the Bureau of Insular Affairs relating to the Philippine Islands located in the U.S. National Archives in College Park, Maryland provided many useful details on U.S. colonial nursing. The court files of Filipina Narciso and Leonora Perez located in the U.S. National Archives in

Chicago contained numerous documents pertaining to the trials of these two women. Finally, the personal collections of individual American and Filipino nurses helped my study tremendously. At a 2000 Asian American History symposium held at the University of California, Los Angeles, an audience member representing an Asian American community organization asked the panelists of an Asian American women's history roundtable (which included myself) what her organization could do to help the research of scholars doing work on Asian American history. I encouraged her and members of her organization to document the history of their organization, collect organizational materials, and secure space for these materials in a library or other venue that would enable researchers to view them. My histories of the Philippine Nurses Association of America (PNAA) and other Filipino nurse organizations would undoubtedly have been enriched by the creation of a public archive of their materials. Although there has been discussion of the creation of such an archival collection at Rutgers University, important historical documents continue to be held by individual PNAA members, some of whom are unwilling to share them with researchers.

During a five-month research trip to the Philippines, I talked with nursing deans, faculty members, and students at several Philippine colleges and schools of nursing in Manila; directors of nursing and staff nurses at private and government hospitals in Manila; the current president and several members of the Philippine Nurses Association; government employees working in overseas-related agencies; and workers in nongovernmental organizations focusing on the welfare of migrant and women workers. My participant-observation included observing a beginning nursing class at Trinity College (formerly St. Luke's Hospital School of Nursing) in Quezon City, Metro Manila (one of the oldest nursing schools in the country), participating in their community health projects and medical missions, and attending nursing and migration conferences.

In Manila, I conducted research in the libraries of Philippine government institutions (such as the Philippine Overseas Employment Administration), nongovernmental institutions (such as Kaibigan for Migrant Workers, Kanlungan Center for Migrant Workers, Center for Women's Resources, and Health Action Information Network), the Philippine Nurses Association, colleges of nursing (such as the University of the Philippines, Philippine Women's University, and De La Salle University), and migration and women's studies centers (such as the Scalabrini Migration Center, St. Scholastica's College Institute of Women's Studies, and the University of the Philippines Center for Women's Studies). These libraries contained Philippine national and international newspaper files on the international migration of Filipino nurses, Philippine nursing journals and texts, government and nongovernmental organization–sponsored international migration studies and statistics, Philippine Nurses Association records, and nursing students' transcript files. In addition, government officers at the Commission on Filipinos Overseas and Commission on Higher Education Development shared recent statistical findings and other documents with me.

Although today it seems that terms like "transnational" have become almost basic elements in American studies vocabulary, during the mid-1990s (when I pursued this research in the Philippines as a doctoral student), my graduate training in American history was defined primarily by scholarship about experiences *within* U.S. national borders, with the exception of the important teaching and guidance I received from Philippine and American historian Michael Salman. Although I do not discuss the details of my Philippine participant-observation and informal interviews in this book, being physically in the Philippines and talking with and observing the activities of various groups and individuals that informed this transnational migrant flow helped me reconceptualize this book from a post-1965 study of Filipino nurses *in* the United States into a study that took seriously the transnational dimensions of this form of migration.

Introduction: The Contours of a Filipino American History

1   Paul Ong and Tania Azores, "The Migration and Incorporation of Filipino Nurses," in *The New Asian Immigration in Los Angeles and Global Restructuring*, ed. Paul Ong, Edna Bonacich, and Lucie Cheng (Philadelphia: Temple University Press, 1994), 164.

2   Ibid., 164, 165.

3   Christine M. Pizer, Ann F. Collard, Christine E. Bishop, Sherline M. James, and Beverly Bonaparte, "Recruiting and Employing Foreign Nurse Graduates in a Large Public Hospital System," *Hospital and Health Services Administration* 39.1 (spring 1994): 17.

4   New York leads these states in employing the majority of foreign nurse graduates. In 1989, it employed 44 percent of this labor force (ibid.).

5   Ong and Azores, "The Migration and Incorporation of Filipino Nurses," 182.

6   According to Ong and Azores, "The proportion of Filipinos who are in the health professions (including doctors and nurses) in Chicago and New York is more than twice that in Los Angeles and more than six times that in San Francisco." See Tania Fortunata Azores-Gunter, "Status Achievement Patterns of Filipinos in the United States" (Ph.D. diss., University of California, Los Angeles, 1987), cited in Ong and Azores, "The Migration and Incorporation of Filipino Nurses," 182.

7   Alfonso Mejía, Helena Pizorkí, and Erica Royston, *Physician and Nurse Migration: Analysis and Policy Implications* (Geneva: World Health Organization, 1979), 43–45.

8   James A. Tyner, "The Global Context of Gendered Labor Migration from the Philippines to the United States," *American Behavioral Scientist* 42.4 (1999): 671.

9   Mejía, Pizorkí, and Royston, *Physician and Nurse Migration: Analysis and Policy Implications*, 47.

10 For example, in their 1992 study, Paul Ong, Lucie Cheng, and Leslie Evans included a number of Asian countries (India, South Korea, Philippines, China, Hong Kong, and Thailand) as well as occupations (math and computer scientists, natural scientists, social scientists, engineers, physicians, nurses, postsecondary teachers) to illustrate the significance of professional migrant flows to the United States and other Western nations. Although the authors did not foreground Filipino nurse migration, their table of immigration of highly educated Asians to the United States between 1972 and 1985 revealed that the number of Filipino nurses (20,482) surpassed those of other Asian highly educated laborers in nine different occupations. Paul M. Ong, Lucie Cheng, and Leslie Evans, "Migration of Highly Educated Asians and Global Dynamics," *Asian and Pacific Migration Journal* 1.3–4 (1992):

543–45. See also Lucie Cheng and Philip Q. Yang, "Global Interaction, Global Inequality, and Migration of the Highly Trained to the United States," *International Migration Review* 32.3 (fall 1998): 626–653, and Wila-wan Kanjanapan, "The Immigration of Asian Professionals to the United States: 1988–1990," *International Migration Review* 29.1 (spring 1995): 7–32. On post-1965 Filipino immigration to the United States, see Benjamin V. Cariño, "The Philippines and Southeast Asia: Historical Roots and Contemporary Linkages," in *Pacific Bridges: The New Immigration from Asia and the Pacific Islands,* ed. James T. Fawcett and Benjamin V. Cariño (Staten Island, N.Y.: Center for Migration Studies, 1987), 305–325; James P. Allen, "Recent Immigration from the Philippines and Filipino Communities in the United States," *Geographical Review* 67.2 (April 1977): 195–208; Peter Smith, "The Social Demography of Filipino Migrations Abroad," *International Migration Review* 10.3 (fall 1976): 307–353; Monica Boyd, "The Changing Nature of Central and Southeast Asian Immigration to the United States: 1961–1972," *International Migration Review* 8.4 (winter 1974): 507–519; Charles B. Keely, "Philippine Migration: International Movement and Immigration to the United States," *International Migration Review* 7.2 (summer 1973): 177–187.

11   See John M. Liu, "The Contours of Asian Professional, Technical and Kindred Work Immigration, 1965–1988," *Sociological Perspectives* 35.4 (1992): 673–704; Justus M. Van Der Kroef, "The U.S. and the World's Brain Drain," *International Journal of Comparative Sociology* 11.3 (1970): 220–239; and Judith A. Fortney, "International Migration of Professionals," *Population Studies* 24 (1970): 217–232.

12   Jon Goss and Bruce Lindquist, "Conceptualizing International Labor Migration: A Structuration Perspective," *International Migration Review* 29.2 (summer 1995): 336.

13   Vicente L. Rafael, *White Love and Other Events in Filipino History* (Durham, NC: Duke University Press, 2000), 23.

14   Michael Salman, "In Our Orientalist Imagination: Historiography and the Culture of Colonialism in the United States," *Radical History Review* 50 (1991): 221–232; Matthew Frye Jacobson, "Imperial Amnesia: Teddy Roosevelt, the Philippines, and the Modern Art of Forgetting," *Radical History Review* 73 (1999): 116–127.

15   See George Lipsitz, *The Possessive Investment in Whiteness: How White People Profit from Identity Politics* (Philadelphia: Temple University Press, 1998), 47–68.

16   See Neil Gotanda, "Comparative Racialization: Racial Profiling and the Case of Wen Ho Lee," *UCLA Law Review* 47 (2000): 1689–1703.

17   Mary Pat Colon, "Why Shouldn't Foreign Nurses Pay Their Own Way?" [letter], *American Journal of Nursing* (October 1978): 1663–1664; emphasis added.

18   Rudolph J. Vecoli, "Comment: We Study the Present to Understand the Past," *Journal of American Ethnic History* 18.4 (summer 1999): 120.

19   In the two major surveys of Asian American history, Takaki's *Strangers from a Different Shore* and Chan's *Asian Americans: An Interpretative History,* Fil-

ipino nurses first emerge in the "post-1965" chapters as a notable Filipino American and professional subgroup. Ronald Takaki, *Strangers from a Different Shore: A History of Asian Americans*, rev. ed. (Boston: Little, Brown, 1998); Sucheng Chan, *Asian Americans: An Interpretive History* (Boston: Twayne Publishers, 1991).

20 Amy Kaplan and Donald Pease, eds., *Cultures of United States Imperialism* (Durham, NC: Duke University Press, 1993); Gilbert M. Joseph, Catherine C. Legrand, and Ricardo D. Salvatore, eds., *Close Encounters of Empire: Writing the Cultural History of U.S.–Latin American Relations* (Durham, NC: Duke University Press, 1998).

21 Alejandro Portes and József Böröcz, "Contemporary Immigration: Theoretical Perspectives on Its Determinants and Modes of Incorporation," *International Migration Review* 23.3–4 (1989): 608.

22 George J. Sánchez, "Race, Nation, and Culture in Recent Immigration Studies," *Journal of American Ethnic History* 18.4 (summer 1999): 75. One noteworthy exception in U.S. immigration historical literature is Matthew Frye Jacobson, *Barbarian Virtues: The United States Encounters Foreign Peoples at Home and Abroad, 1876–1917* (New York: Hill and Wang, 2000). However, Jacobson is less concerned about the ways U.S. imperialism abroad produces specific colonial migrations; rather, he focuses on the way "immigration and expansionism constituted two sides of the same coin" during the late nineteenth and early twentieth centuries as products of the "same economic engines of industrialization" and as part of the "national debate over the 'fitness for self-government' of problematic peoples abroad" (4).

23 Paul Ong, Edna Bonacich, and Lucie Cheng, "The Political Economy of Capitalist Restructuring and the New Asian Immigration," in *The New Asian Immigration in Los Angeles and Global Restructuring*, ed. Ong, Bonacich, and Cheng, 4.

24 David M. Reimers, *Still the Golden Door: The Third World Comes to America*, 2d ed. (New York: Columbia University Press, 1992), 93.

25 Karen Brodkin Sacks and Nancy Scheper-Hughes, "Introduction," *Women's Studies* 13 (1987): 176.

26 Ong, Cheng, and Evans, "Migration of Highly Educated Asians and Global Dynamics," 543.

27 Darlene Clark Hine, *Black Women in White: Racial Conflict and Cooperation in the Nursing Profession, 1890–1950* (Bloomington: Indiana University Press, 1989).

28 John Carlos Rowe, ed., *Post-Nationalist American Studies* (Berkeley: University of California Press, 2000).

29 For a critical analysis of these changes in the field of Asian American studies, see Sau-Ling Wong, "Denationalization Reconsidered: Asian American Cultural Criticism at a Theoretical Crossroads," *Amerasia Journal* 21.1–2 (1995): 1–27.

30 Madeline Hsu, *Dreaming of Gold, Dreaming of Home: Transnationalism and Migration between the United States and South China, 1882–1943* (Stanford, CA: Stanford University Press, 2000).

31   See Chan, *Asian Americans;* Gary Okihiro, *Common Ground: Reimaging American History* (Princeton, NJ: Princeton University Press, 2001), and *Margins and Mainstreams: Asians in American History and Culture* (Seattle: University of Washington Press, 1994); Ronald Takaki, *A Different Mirror: A History of Multicultural America* (Boston: Little, Brown, 1993), and *Strangers from a Different Shore.*

32   Sucheng Chan, "Asian American Historiography," *Pacific Historical Review* 35 (1996): 397.

33   Jacobson, "Imperial Amnesia: Teddy Roosevelt, the Philippines, and the Modern Art of Forgetting."

34   Jesse Ventura, *I Ain't Got Time to Bleed: Reworking the Body Politic from the Bottom Up* (New York: Villard, 1999), 78–79.

35   Catherine Ceniza Choy, "Asian American History: Reflections on Imperialism, Immigration, and 'The Body,'" *Amerasia Journal* 26.1 (2000): 119–140.

36   H. Brett Melendy, *Asians in America: Filipinos, Koreans, and East Indians* (Boston: Twayne Publishers, 1977), 96, as cited in Yen Le Espiritu, "Colonial Oppression, Labour Importation, and Group Formation: Filipinos in the United States," *Ethnic and Racial Studies* 19.1 (January 1996): 37.

37   Philippine Study Group of Minnesota, "Philippine Study Group of Minnesota Corrects the Misleading Philippine American War Plaque at the Minnesota State Capitol," Internet online, accessed 22 February 2002. Available from http://www.crcworks.org/plaque.html.

1. Nursing Matters: Women and U.S.
Colonialism in the Philippines

1   Patrocinio J. Montellano, "Years That Count," *Philippine Journal of Nursing* [hereafter *PJN*] 31.4 (July–August 1962): 235.

2   Jose P. Bantug, *A Short History of Medicine in the Philippines during the Spanish Regime, 1565–1898* (Manila: Colegio Médico-Farmacéutico de Filipinas, 1953), 126.

3   For an overview of the history of ilustrados, see Renato Constantino, *The Philippines: A Past Revisited* (Manila: Renato Constantino, 1975); John N. Schumacher, *The Propaganda Movement 1880–1895: The Creators of a Filipino Consciousness, the Makers of Revolution* (Manila: Ateneo de Manila University Press, 1997).

4   For example, Elizabeth Uy Eviota claims that "American policy in ruling also did not differ much from Spain. . . . As in Spanish colonial policy, American political administration had no place for women." Elizabeth Uy Eviota, *The Political Economy of Gender: Women and the Sexual Division of Labor in the Philippines* (London: Zed Books, 1992), 63.

5   Montellano, "Years That Count," 235.

6   The following anthologies provide a broad spectrum of new scholarly production in the field of women and imperialism: Antionette Burton, ed., *Gender, Sexuality and Colonial Modernities* (New York: Routledge, 1999);

Ruth Roach Pierson and Nupur Chaudhuri, eds., *Nation, Empire, Colony: Historicizing Gender and Race* (Bloomington: Indiana University Press, 1998); Nupur Chaudhuri and Margaret Strobel, eds., *Western Women and Imperialism: Complicity and Resistance* (Bloomington: Indiana University Press, 1992).

7   Recent works that challenge the invisibility of American women's roles in U.S. imperialism in the Philippines are Vicente L. Rafael's chapter "Colonial Domesticity: Engendering Race at the Edge of Empire, 1899–1912," in *White Love and Other Events in Filipino History* (Durham, NC: Duke University Press, 2000), 52–75; Laura Wexler, *Tender Violence: Domestic Visions in an Age of U.S. Imperialism* (Chapel Hill: University of North Carolina Press, 2000); Louise Michele Newman, *White Women's Rights: The Racial Origins of Feminism in the United States* (New York: Oxford University Press, 1999).

8   Reynaldo C. Ileto, "Cholera and the Origins of the American Sanitary Order in the Philippines," in *Discrepant Histories: Translocal Essays on Filipino Cultures*, ed. Vicente L. Rafael (Manila: Anvil Publishing, 1995), 51.

9   For an overview of this historiographical shift and trends and gaps in this scholarly field, see Shula Marks, "What Is Colonial about Colonial Medicine? And What Has Happened to Imperialism and Health?" *Society for the Social History of Medicine* 10.2 (1997): 205–219. The following anthologies offer a range of scholarly works that represent this shift: Roy MacLeod and Milton Lewis, eds., *Disease, Medicine, and Empire: Perspectives on Western Medicine and the Experience of European Expansion* (London: Routledge, 1988); Teresa Meade and Mark Walker, eds., *Science, Medicine, and Cultural Imperialism* (New York: St. Martin's Press, 1991).

10 The classic account of these Filipino male migrant workers' experiences is Carlos Bulosan's *America Is in the Heart* (New York: Harcourt, Brace and Company, 1943). See also Chapter 9 in Ronald Takaki, *Strangers from a Different Shore: A History of Asian Americans,* rev. ed. (Boston: Little, Brown, 1998), 315–354. For a history of Asian American laborers, including Filipino laborers, in the Northwest canneries, see Chris Friday, *Organizing Asian American Labor: The Pacific Coast Canned-Salmon Industry, 1870–1942* (Philadelphia: Temple University Press, 1994). For a history of Asian American laborers, including Filipino laborers, in Hawaiian plantations, see Ronald Takaki, *Pau Hana: Plantation Life and Labor in Hawaii* (Honolulu: University of Hawai'i Press, 1983).

11 Victor G. Heiser, "Unsolved Health Problems Peculiar to the Philippines," *Philippine Journal of Science* 5.2 (July 1910): 177, in Record Group [hereafter RG] 350, Box 275, File 2394-25, U.S. National Archives, College Park, Maryland (hereafter USNA).

12 Quoted in Constantino, *The Philippines: A Past Revisited,* 223.

13 Heiser, "Unsolved Health Problems Peculiar to the Philippines," 177–178.

14 Jean Comaroff, "The Diseased Heart of Africa: Medicine, Colonialism, and the Black Body," in *Knowledge, Power and Practice: The Anthropology of Medicine and Everyday Life,* ed. Shirley Lindenbaum and Margaret Lock (Berkeley: University of California Press, 1993), 313.

15 Ileto, "Cholera and the Origins of the American Sanitary Order in the Philippines," 60–61.

16 David Arnold, *Colonizing the Body: State Medicine and Epidemic Disease in Nineteenth Century India* (Berkeley: University of California Press, 1993), 89.

17 Quoted in Warwick Anderson, "'Where Every Prospect Pleases and Only Man Is Vile,'" in *Discrepant Histories: Translocal Essays on Filipino Cultures,* ed. Vicente L. Rafael (Manila: Anvil Publishing, 1995), 100.

18 According to Hindu beliefs, smallpox was not a disease but the presence of the goddess Sitala. Hindus employed religious rituals to appease the goddess. Another Indian method of controlling smallpox was variolation, inoculation with live smallpox matter to produce a moderated form of the disease and to protect the individual from future outbreaks (Arnold, *Colonizing the Body,* 120).

19 Ibid., 137.

20 Ileto, "Cholera and the Origins of the American Sanitary Order in the Philippines," 58.

21 See Anastacia Girón-Tupas, *History of Nursing in the Philippines* (Manila: University Book Supply, 1952), 28.

22 See Dea Birkett, "The 'White Women's Burden' in the 'White Man's Grave': The Introduction of British Nurses in Colonial West Africa," in *Western Women and Imperialism: Complicity and Resistance,* ed. Chaudhuri and Strobel, 177–188; Helen Callaway's chapter "Women in Health Care" in *Gender, Culture and Empire: European Women in Colonial Nigeria* (Urbana: University of Illinois Press, 1987), 83–109.

23 According to Louise Newman, late nineteenth- and early twentieth-century white American women's rights activists conceived assimilation and civilizing missions as "humane alternatives to the violence and coercion that male politicians had condoned in whites' dealing with the so-called primitive groups of Indians, Chinese, Africans and Filipinos" (Newman, *White Women's Rights,* 182).

24 Lavinia L. Dock, "Lavinia L. Dock: Self-Portrait, July 6, 1931," cited in Mary Ann Bradford Burnam, "Lavinia Lloyd Dock: An Activist in Nursing and Social Reform" (Ph.D. diss., Ohio State University, 1998), 274.

25 Rafael, *White Love and Other Events in Filipino History,* 54.

26 Ileto, "Cholera and the Origins of the American Sanitary Order in the Philippines," 61–62.

27 Lavinia L. Dock, *A History of Nursing: From the Earliest Times to the Present Day with Special Reference to the Work of the Past Thirty Years* (New York: Putnam's, 1912), 4:311.

28 Ibid., 317.

29 Ibid., 313–314.

30 Ileto, "Cholera and the Origins of the American Sanitary Order in the Philippines," 63.

31 Dock, *A History of Nursing,* 314.

32 Newman, *White Women's Rights,* 34.

33   Dock, *A History of Nursing*, 315.

34   Ibid., 310–311; emphasis added.

35   Anderson, "'Where Every Prospect Pleases and Only Man Is Vile,'" 84, 95–99.

36   Susan M. Reverby, *Ordered to Care: The Dilemma of American Nursing, 1850–1945* (Cambridge, England: Cambridge University Press, 1987), 24.

37   "Extract from letter of March 18, 1902 from P.I. Civil Service Board to U.S. Civ. Ser. Comm'n and transmitted by them Apr. 24, 1902," RG 350, Box 407, File 5235, USNA. See also Victor G. Heiser to the Acting Secretary of the Interior, January 29, 1907, RG 350, Box 407, File 5235-36, USNA.

38   W. S. Washburn to U.S. Civil Service Commission, October 29, 1903, RG 350, Box 407, File 5235, USNA.

39   See Kelvin A. Santiago-Valles, "'Higher Womanhood' among the 'Lower Races': Julia McNair Henry in Puerto Rico and the 'Burdens' of 1898," *Radical History Review* 73 (1999): 48.

40   Rafael, *White Love and Other Events in Filipino History*, 58.

41   "Trained Nurse: Philippine Service," August 22, 1911, RG 350, Box 407, File 5235-134, USNA.

42   Mabel E. McCalmont to Superintendent, Training School for Nurses, March 11, 1909, RG 350, Box 407, File 5235-77, USNA.

43   See Mary Louise Pratt, *Imperial Eyes: Travel Writing and Transculturation* (New York: Routledge, 1992), 5.

44   Miscellaneous news excerpts from the P.I. Civil Service Commission, RG 350, Box 407, File 5235, USNA; Frank McIntyre to War Department, Bureau of Insular Affairs, October 24, 1906, RG 350, Box 407, File 5235-26, USNA.

45   Victor G. Heiser to Major McIntyre, February 7, 1910, RG 350, Box 407, File 5235-87, USNA.

46   Mabel E. McCalmont to Major McIntyre, February 4, 1910, p. 2, RG 350, Box 407, File 5235-88, USNA.

47   Alice Louise Bruton to Frank McIntyre, September 30, 1913, p. 7, RG 350, Box 330, File 3267-34, USNA.

48   Mary J. Dugan to Frank McIntyre, September 30, 1913, p. 1, RG 350, Box 330, File 3267-35, USNA.

49   As Louise Newman writes, "By offering themselves as the epitome of social evolutionary development, [white American women] were also trying, simultaneously, if paradoxically, to articulate an egalitarian vision, one that could be inclusive of women of color and that envisioned 'lower races' as their potential equals *in the future*" (Newman, *White Women's Rights*, 20; emphasis in original).

50   *Philippine General Hospital School of Nursing Ninth Annual Announcement and Catalogue, 1915–1916*, p. 14, RG 350, Box 967, File 21553-16, USNA.

51   Quoted in Girón-Tupas, *History of Nursing in the Philippines*, 41.

52   As Paul Kramer argues, "The Philippine Scouts were brought to the fair to illustrate the process of Filipino 'evolution' under American colonial 'tutelage,' their discipline and American traits held in contrast to more 'backward' groups." Paul Kramer, "Making Concessions: Race and Empire Re-

visited at the Philippine Exposition, St. Louis, 1901–1905," *Radical History Review* 73 (1999): 99.

53 Quoted in Girón-Tupas, *History of Nursing in the Philippines,* 42.

54 Quoted in Julita Villaruel Sotejo and Mary Vita G. Beltran-Jackson, *Learning Nursing at the Bedside: Nursing Education Practices—Past and Present,* 2d ed. (Quezon City: University of the Philippines Press, 1965), 18.

55 There are numerous examples of this pattern: founder and Dean of the University of the Philippines College of Nursing Julita Sotejo received her M.S. from the University of Chicago; University of the Philippines College of Nursing Professor Amelia Mangay Maglacas received her M.S. from University of Minnesota; St. Luke's Hospital School of Nursing Principal Ester Santos received her B.S.N. from Columbia University.

56 For a description of the original pensionado movement, see William Alexander Sutherland, *Not by Might: The Epic of the Philippines* (Las Cruces, NM: Southwest Publishing, 1953).

57 Montellano, "Years That Count," 235.

58 "What Our Women Are Studying," *Filipino Student Bulletin, Special Filipino Women Students' Number* 5.8 (April–May 1926):1, in Filipino American National Historical Society Archives, Seattle, WA.

59 D. B. Ambrosio, "Filipino Women in U.S. Excel in Their Courses: Invade Business, Politics," *Filipino Student Bulletin, Special Filipino Women Students' Number* 5.8 (April–May 1926): 1–2, in Filipino American National Historical Society Archives, Seattle, WA.

60 Quoted in Barbara L. Brush, "The Rockefeller Agenda for American/Philippine Nursing Relations," *Western Journal of Nursing Research* 17.5 (1995): 545, 549, 548.

61 Elsie P. McCloskey to Brigadier General McIntyre, May 29, 1915, RG 350, Box 967, File 21553-17, USNA.

62 Emma Sarepta Yule, "Filipino Feminism," *Scribner's* (June 1920): 737, 743, in RG 350, Box 871, File 17087-6, USNA.

63 Dock, *A History of Nursing,* 313–314.

64 Joan Jacobs Brumberg, "Zenanas and Girlless Villages: The Ethnology of American Evangelical Women, 1870–1910," *Journal of American History* 69 (September 1982): 349, cited in Newman, *White Women's Rights,* 7.

65 Encarnacion Alzona, *The Filipino Woman: Her Social, Economic, and Political Status, 1565–1933* (Manila: University of the Philippines Press, 1934), 3, 15–16, 53–54.

66 Paz Policarpio Mendez, "The Progress of the Filipino Woman during the Last Sixty Years," paper prepared for the 60th anniversary of the First Feminist Movement in the Philippines, Centro Escolar University in the Philippines, 12 August 1965, 2; emphasis added.

67 Alzona, *The Filipino Woman,* 18–19.

68 Encarnacion Alzona, *The Filipino Woman: Her Social, Economic, and Political Status, 1565–1937,* rev. ed. (Manila: Benipayo Press, 1938), 123.

69 W. W. Marquardt, "Applications for Nursing Positions," June 19, 1916, RG 350, Box 968, File 21553-20, USNA.

70   W. E. Musgrave to W. W. Marquardt, January 12, 1921, RG 350, Box 576, File 5235-164, USNA.

71   W. W. Marquardt to W. E. Musgrave, January 19, 1921, RG 350, Box 576, File 5235-164, USNA; emphasis added.

72   Maria Abastilla Beltran, interview by Carolina Koslosky, tape recording, Seattle, WA, 5 May 1975, for Demonstration Project for Asian Americans, in Filipino American National Historical Society Archives, Seattle, WA.

2. "The Usual Subjects": The Preconditions of
Professional Migration

1   Lavinia L. Dock, *A History of Nursing: From the Earliest Times to the Present Day with Special Reference to the Work of the Past Thirty Years* (New York: Putnam's, 1912), 4: 316; emphasis added.

2   See Paul Ong and Tania Azores, "The Migration and Incorporation of Filipino Nurses," in *The New Asian Immigration in Los Angeles and Global Restructuring,* ed. Paul Ong, Edna Bonacich, and Lucie Cheng (Philadelphia: Temple University Press, 1994), 164–195; Tomoji Ishi, "Class Conflict, the State, and Linkage: The International Migration of Nurses from the Philippines," *Berkeley Journal of Sociology* 32 (1987): 281–312.

3   Antoinette Burton uses this phrase to problematize and qualify the power of modern colonizing regimes. Antoinette Burton, "The Unfinished Business of Colonial Modernities," in *Gender, Sexuality and Colonial Modernities,* ed. Antoinette Burton (New York: Routledge, 1999), 1.

4   *Philippine General Hospital School of Nursing Ninth Annual Announcement and Catalogue, 1915–1916,* p. 19, RG 350, Box 967, File 21553-16, USNA.

5   This strategy changed, however, in the 1830s. David Arnold, *Colonizing the Body: State Medicine and Epidemic Disease in Nineteenth Century India* (Berkeley: University of California Press, 1993), 54–55.

6   Rita Headrick, *Colonialism, Health and Illness in French Equatorial Africa, 1885–1935* (Atlanta, GA: African Studies Association Press, 1994), 245, 252–253.

7   *Philippine General Hospital School of Nursing Ninth Annual Announcement and Catalogue, 1915–1916,* p. 20.

8   The Government of the Philippine Islands, Department of the Interior, Board of Examiners for Nurses, Manila, "Rules of the Board of Examiners for Nurses," May 7, 1920, p. 12, RG 350, Box 967, File 21553-37, USNA.

9   "An Act to Provide for the Establishment of Class for Training in Nursing in the Philippine Normal School, and Appropriating the Sum of Twenty Thousand Pesos for Such Purpose," May 20, 1909, RG 350, Box 407, File 5235-75, USNA.

10 Susan M. Reverby, *Ordered to Care: The Dilemma of American Nursing, 1850–1945* (Cambridge, England: Cambridge University Press, 1987), 15–20, 27, 39–47.

11 Anastacia Girón-Tupas, *History of Nursing in the Philippines* (Manila: University Book Supply, 1952), 62.

12 Reverby, *Ordered to Care*, 48.

13 Ibid., 84.

14 For example, Ramona Cabrera, one of the first graduates of the Philippine General Hospital School of Nursing, moved from Cebu to study at the school in Manila (Girón-Tupas, *History of Nursing in the Philippines*, 42).

15 Ibid., 39. This type of learning would later be incorporated into the curriculum of schools of nursing in courses such as etiquette, which was a "combined lecture and demonstration course in personal, social, and hospital etiquette." *Philippine General Hospital School of Nursing Ninth Annual Announcement and Catalogue, 1915–1916*, p. 20.

16 Girón-Tupas, *History of Nursing in the Philippines*, 34; emphasis added.

17 Barbara Melosh, *"The Physician's Hand": Work Culture and Conflict in American Nursing* (Philadelphia: Temple University Press, 1982), 37. Girón-Tupas writes that the earliest schools of nursing required that the students reside in the dormitory for Filipino women. In my interviews with Filipino nurses, those nurses who studied in hospital schools of nursing were also required to live in the hospital nursing residence.

18 Interview with Purita Asperilla, November 11, 1994, New York, NY.

19 See Reverby, *Ordered to Care*, 60–76.

20 Interview with Purita Asperilla.

21 *Philippine General Hospital School of Nursing Ninth Annual Announcement and Catalogue, 1915–1916*, pp. 20, 17.

22 Ibid., 13; emphasis added.

23 Ibid., 37–44.

24 *Philippine General Hospital School of Nursing Tenth Annual Announcement and Catalogue, 1916–1917*, pp. 3, 9, RG 350, Box 968, File 21553-19, USNA.

25 *Philippine General Hospital School of Nursing Ninth Annual Announcement and Catalogue, 1915–1916*, pp. 15, 18; emphasis added.

26 Daisy Caroline Bridges, *A History of the International Council of Nurses, 1899–1964: The First Sixty-Five Years* (Philadelphia: Lippincott, 1967), 38.

27 Quoted in Barbara L. Brush, "The Rockefeller Agenda for American/Philippine Nursing Relations," *Western Journal of Nursing Research* 17.5 (1995): 550.

28 *Philippine General Hospital School of Nursing Tenth Annual Announcement and Catalogue, 1916–1917*, p. 9.

29 *Manual for Nurses of the Philippine General Hospital*, 1923, p. 212, RG 350, Box 968, File 21553-36, USNA; emphasis added.

30 Brush, "The Rockefeller Agenda for American/Philippine Nursing Relations," 550.

31 See Reverby, *Ordered to Care*, 121–142; Melosh, *"The Physician's Hand,"* 33–34.

32 Girón-Tupas, *History of Nursing in the Philippines*, 40.

33 Ibid., 63.

34 See Melosh, "Public-Health Nurses and the 'Gospel of Health,' 1920–1955," in *"The Physician's Hand."*

35 See Soledad A. Buenafe, "Some Highlights in the Development of Public

Health Nursing in the Bureau of Health," *PJN* 41.3 (July–September 1972): 115–120.

36 Director of Health to Issabella Waters, June 10, 1915, with attachments of "Information Desired," RG 350, Box 576, File 5235-161, USNA.

37 Interview with Purita Asperilla.

38 Girón-Tupas, *History of Nursing in the Philippines,* 104–105.

39 Soledad A. Buenafe and Patrocinio J. Montellano, "Forty Years of the Filipino Nurses' Association," *PJN* 31.5 (September–October 1962): 299–312, 348.

40 Ibid., 299.

41 Ibid., 300.

42 Julita Villaruel Sotejo and Mary Vita G. Beltran-Jackson, *Learning Nursing at the Bedside: Nursing Education Practices — Past and Present,* 2d ed. (Quezon City, Metro Manila: S. J. Publications, 1972), 43–74.

43 Bridges, *A History of the International Council of Nurses,* 230, 55, 75–76.

44 Ibid., 89.

45 Interview with Josefina R. Sablan, May 10, 1995, New York, NY.

46 Girón-Tupas, *History of Nursing in the Philippines,* 44–45.

47 These programs included University of Santo Tomas School of Nursing Education, University of the Philippines College of Nursing, Manila Central University College of Nursing, Philippine Union College, Central Philippines College, St. Paul's School of Nursing, Silliman University, Philippine Women's University, and Southwestern College of Nursing. For a brief overview of these programs, see Girón-Tupas, *History of Nursing in the Philippines,* 109–116.

48 This pattern continued through the 1950s. Rosario T. Degracia studied at Case Western University in 1957 also under the auspices of a China Medical Board fellowship. Interview with Rosario T. Degracia, December 14, 1994, Seattle, WA.

49 Interview with Purita Asperilla.

3. "Your Cap Is a Passport": Filipino Nurses and the U.S. Exchange Visitor Program

1 Interview with Epifania O. Mercado, February 3, 1995, New York, NY.

2 U.S. Congress, Senate, "Promoting the Better Understanding of the United States among the Peoples of the World and to Strengthen Cooperative International Relations," S. Rpt. 811, 80th Congress, 2d sess., *Senate Miscellaneous Reports I* (Washington, DC: Government Printing Office, 1948), 4.

3 The ANA made second, or subsequent, placements for American exchange visitor nurses already abroad. The statistics I analyze here refer to new exchange visitor arrangements only. The ANA did not publish statistics on American exchange nurses abroad before 1957 in *Facts about Nursing.* Of the seventy-six American exchange nurses, thirty-one visited Great Britain and fifteen visited Denmark. The remaining American exchange nurses primarily visited other Northern European countries: France (9), Sweden (4), Ger-

many (3), Switzerland (3), Holland (2), Norway (1), Finland (1), and Scotland (1). Exceptions during this period include six American exchange nurse arrangements in Haiti, India, and South Africa. See ANA Nursing Information Bureau, *Facts about Nursing* (New York: American Nurses Association, 1959–1961).

4   According to Barbara Brush, between 1949 and 1951, Danish nurses constituted 54 percent of exchangees, Swedish nurses 11 percent, British nurses 9 percent, and Norwegian nurses 6 percent. She cites statistics compiled from a 1951 report, "Study Programs and Employment Arranged for Foreign Nurses Who Are Present in the U.S.A.," from the ANA Collection at the nursing archives in Boston University Mugar Library. She does not indicate the total number of exchange visitors in the United States during this period from which the percentages have been calculated. It is also unclear whether the numbers of exchange visitor nurses she is referring to are those sponsored by the ANA only or those sponsored by all U.S. organizations and institutions. See Barbara Brush, " 'Exchangees' or Employees?" *Nursing History Review* 1.1 (1993): 173, 179. This trend continued in the late 1950s with the number of ANA-sponsored Danish, Swedish, and British exchange nurses continuing to surpass the number of exchange nurses from the Philippines. The ANA did not publish statistics on foreign exchange nurses in the United States before 1956 in *Facts about Nursing*. In the late 1950s, the number of exchange nurses from Australia and the Philippines became noteworthy as well, while those from Norway became less significant over time. During this period, Australia sent the highest number (159) of new ANA-sponsored exchange visitor nurses (961 total). The number of exchange visitor nurses from Denmark (115), Great Britain (89), and Sweden (80) surpassed those from the Philippines (77).

5   Although the EVP began in 1948, it was not until 1951 that the Filipino Nurses Association began assisting Filipino nurses with exchange arrangements. Philippine President Ramon Magsaysay created an Exchange Visitor Program Committee only in 1956 to screen applicants.

6   Purita Falgui Asperilla, "The Mobility of Filipino Nurses" (Ph.D. diss., Columbia University, 1971), 5, 53. Between 1956 and 1969, nurses constituted over 50 percent (11,136) of the total number (20,420) of exchange visitors from the Philippines. While nurses made up the largest occupational group among Filipino EVP participants, health personnel in general dominated Filipino participation in the program. From 1956 to 1969, 6,250 Filipino exchange visitors were physicians. Purificacion Capulong's study of the EVP supports Asperilla's findings regarding the numerical domination of nurses specifically, and health personnel in general, among Filipino EVP participants. Between 1956 and 1964, Capulong notes that out of a total of 9,592 Filipino exchange visitors, 5,708 were nurses, 3,556 were physicians, 979 were medical technologists, 190 were dietitians, and 95 were dentists. See Purificacion N. Capulong, "An Appraisal of the United States Exchange-Visitor Program for Filipino Nurses" (M.A. thesis, Philippine Women's University, 1965), 12–13, 152.

7 Tomoji Ishi, "Class Conflict, the State, and Linkage: The International Migration of Nurses from the Philippines," *Berkeley Journal of Sociology* 32 (1987): 290. In 1966, 1,364 of a total of 1,817 exchange visitor nurses admitted to the United States came from the Philippines. This numerical dominance continued over the next two years, with Filipino exchange nurses constituting 1,194 of 1,603 exchange nurses in 1967, and 1,095 of 1,485 in 1968. Although the 162 exchange nurses from Korea and 86 exchange nurses from the United Kingdom admitted to the United States between 1966 and 1968 outnumbered those from other countries, their numbers appear almost insignificant when compared to the several thousands of exchange nurses from the Philippines.

8 Martha Jeanne Broadhurst, "Knowing Our Exchange Visitors," *Nursing Outlook* 6 (April 1958): 201.

9 "Local News: 104 Young Nurses Off to U.S.," *PJN* 29.3 (May–June 1960): 195–196; "Local News: 122 Young Nurses Departed to U.S.," *PJN* 29.4 (July–August, 1960): 267–268.

10 J. C. Bacala, "This Issue's Personality: Juanita J. Jimenez, a Silver Lining in Our Profession," *PJN* 31.3 (May–June 1962): 192–193.

11 Smith Bell & Co. Travel & Tours Department advertisement, *PJN* 35.5 (September–October 1966).

12 Commercial Credit Corporation of Greater Manila Travel Department advertisement, *PJN* 35.5 (September–October 1966); emphasis added.

13 Interview with Milagros Rabara, March 21, 1995, New York, NY.

14 Interview with Lourdes Velasco, February 6, 1995, New York, NY.

15 Interview with Hermila M. Rabe, January 27, 1995, New York, NY.

16 Alfredo S. Quijano, "No Brain Drain, but There Is No Job Opportunity Here for Nurses," *Examiner,* 9 November 1968, p. 8.

17 According to the Bureau of Labor Statistics in 1966, general duty nurses in the United States earned a weekly average of $100.50. In 1969, an ANA study found that staff nurses in the United States earned a weekly average of $133. ANA Nursing Information Bureau, *Facts about Nursing* (New York: American Nurses Association, 1969), 124.

18 Interview with Luz Alerta, March 13, 1995, New York, NY.

19 Interview with Josephine Abalos, March 18, 1995, New York, NY.

20 Interview with Ofelia Boado, February 6, 1995, New York, NY.

21 Ibid.

22 Asperilla, "The Mobility of Filipino Nurses," 43–44.

23 Interview with Ofelia Boado.

24 Ibid.

25 Ibid.

26 Interview with Julieta Luistro, April 25, 1995, New York, NY. Luistro returned to the Philippines in 1966; she married her boyfriend in 1968.

27 Gary Hawes, *The Philippine State and the Marcos Regime: The Politics of Export* (Ithaca, NY: Cornell University Press, 1987), 27–28.

28 Vicente L. Rafael, *White Love and Other Events in Filipino History* (Durham, NC: Duke University Press, 2000), 260.

29 Interview with Julieta Luistro.

30 Interview with Milagros Rabara.

31 Interview with Josephine Abalos.

32 Tomas Antonio de la Vaca, "Should Filipino Students Take Their Basic Nursing Studies Abroad?" *Santo Tomas Nursing Journal* 1.3 (December 1962): 183.

33 Luisa A. Alvarez, "The President's Page: Words to Student Nurses," *PJN* 32.4 (July–August 1963): 169.

34 St. Luke's College of Nursing, Trinity College, Quezon City, Philippines, transcript files. There were many other applicants who mentioned goals of "going abroad" in general, though not specifically through the EVP. I was unable to conduct a more systematic study of these student records, as the transcript files were in the process of being reorganized during my research visit.

35 Asperilla, "The Mobility of Filipino Nurses," 15–17, 72.

36 Interview with Milagros Rabara.

37 Teodora Ignacio, Marlena Masaganda, and Leticia Sta. Maria, "A Study of the Graduates of the Basic Degree Program of the University of the Philippines College of Nursing Who Have Gone Abroad," *ANPHI* (October 1967): 50–68.

38 According to the FNA, "since 1951, when the FNA started sending nurses under the Exchange Visitor Program thru [*sic*] the American Nurses Association, there was not a single complaint coming from Filipino nurses sponsored by the ANA." "Ed. Note," *PJN* 32.1 (January–February 1963): 6.

39 According to Purificacion Capulong, from 1956 to 1964, 5,708 Filipino nurses participated in the exchange program. Yet, from 1948 to 1964, the FNA coordinated the placement of only 122 Filipino exchange nurses (Capulong, "Appraisal of the United States Exchange-Visitor Program," 77). Furthermore, the FNA was unable to coordinate placement of the maximum number of Filipino exchange nurse openings allotted by the ANA. According to Capulong, as the ANA processed exchange nurse applications from all over the world, it accepted a maximum of 48 nurses from the Philippines annually for sponsorship. Because the FNA began coordinating placements of Filipino exchange nurses in 1951, they would have been able to facilitate the placement of up to 672 nurses from the Philippines between 1951 and 1964. Having placed only 122 during this period, the FNA utilized under 20 percent of the available ANA exchange openings. Asperilla's study suggests that the majority of Filipino exchange nurses arranged placements directly with sponsoring hospitals (Asperilla, "The Mobility of Filipino Nurses," 141).

40 Miguela Z. Tena, "The Nurses and the Nursing Profession," *PJN* 29.4 (July–August 1960): 241.

41 A Group of Young Graduates to the Editor, "From the Mail Box," *PJN* 29.5 (September–October 1960): 270.

42 Philippine Air Lines advertisement, *PJN* 33.5 (September–October 1964); Northwest Air Lines advertisement, *PJN* 38.3 (July–September 1969).

43 Interview with Lourdes Velasco.

44 J. C. Bacala, "The Trouble with Our Exchange Visitor Nurses," *PJN* 32.3 (May–June 1963): 142.

45 Continental Tours advertisement, *PJN* 35.5 (September–October 1966).

46 See Epifanio B. Castillejos, "The Exchange Visitors Program: Report and Recommendation," *PJN* 35.5 (September–October 1966): 306–307.

47 Interview with Josephine Abalos.

48 Interview with Christina B. Hing, February 7, 1995, New York, NY.

49 Fortunata T. Kennedy, letter to the author, 27 February 1995.

50 Interview with Lourdes Velasco.

51 Using Filipino exchange nurses as nurse's aides was one of many abuses of the EVP, according to some Filipino exchange nurse returnees. See Patria G. Alinea and Gloria B. Senador, "Leaving for Abroad? . . . Here's a Word of Caution," *PJN* 42.1 (January–March 1973): 92–94.

52 Interview with Josephine Abalos.

53 In 1946, the director of the Nursing Information Bureau reported that the American health care system required 41,700 additional nurses. The demand for nursing care was particularly acute in U.S. hospitals, which in 1946 admitted one million more patients than the previous year. See Mary Roberts, preface to *Facts about Nursing* by ANA Nursing Information Bureau (New York: American Nurses Association, 1946), 3. By 1951, the president of the ANA estimated that current civilian nursing needs required 65,000 additional nurses. See Elizabeth K. Porter, preface to *Facts about Nursing* by ANA Nursing Information Bureau (New York: American Nurses Association, 1951), 3.

54 ANA Nursing Information Bureau, *Facts about Nursing* (New York: American Nurses Association, 1962–1963), 28; ANA Nursing Information Bureau, *Facts about Nursing* (New York: American Nurses Association, 1961). A comparative and statistical overview of exchange nurse stipends and U.S. general duty nurse earnings necessitates further research.

55 "Filipino Nurses Win Case: Hospital Coordinator Resigned," *PJN* 36.4 (July–August 1967): 230.

56 Filipino exchange nurses in Galveston were not the only nurses to organize a PNA chapter in the United States and to seek recognition as a chapter abroad during this period. I discuss these other organizations in more detail in Chapter 6. In this chapter, I use the terms FNA and PNA interchangeably.

57 Yolanda Fabros to Secretary, Filipino Nurses Association, "In Our Mail," *PJN* 34.5 (September–October 1965): 254.

58 Interview with Luzviminda Micabalo, November 16, 1994, New York, NY.

59 Capulong, "Appraisal of the United States Exchange-Visitor Program," 81–82.

60 American Nurses Association, "ANA Statement on the Practices Relating to Nurses from Abroad," *PJN* 29.2 (March–April 1960): 58–59.

61 Study Committee of the Department of Labor, the Philippines, *Report on the Problem of Brain Drain in the Philippines* (Manila: Philippine Department of Labor, 1966), 2, cited in Asperilla, "The Mobility of Filipino Nurses," 54.

62 Interview with Priscilla Santayana, November 19, 1994, New York, NY.

63   Castillejos, "The Exchange Visitors Program," 306–307.

64   Interview with Lourdes Velasco.

65   Asperilla, "The Mobility of Filipino Nurses," 52. According to Asperilla, between 1967 and 1970, 3,279 Filipino nurses left the Philippines through the EVP.

66   Luisa A. Alvarez, "By the President," *PJN* 29.3 (May–June 1960): 133.

67   *Lilia B. Velasco v. Immigration and Naturalization Service, Nellie J. C. Morales v. Immigration and Naturalization Service*, 386 F.2d 283 (1967).

68   Ibid., 286.

69   *Marina E. Alonzo v. Immigration and Naturalization Service*, 408 F.2d 667 (1969), 667, 668.

70   "The Filipino Nurses' Hymn," *PJN* 31.1 (January–February 1962): 34.

71   Pura S. Castrence, "Challenge to the Filipino Nurses," *PJN* 35.4 (July–August 1966): 207.

72   Paulino J. Garcia, "The Sense of Mission in Nursing and the Temptations against It," *PJN* 34.2 (March–April 1965): 70–71.

73   Ibid., 70.

74   Castrence, "Challenge to the Filipino Nurses," 207.

75   Garcia, "The Sense of Mission in Nursing and the Temptations against It," 70.

76   Castrence, "Challenge to the Filipino Nurses," 206–207.

77   Asperilla, "The Mobility of Filipino Nurses," 151. In Asperilla's study of 411 Filipino nurse returnees, 97 percent said they would like to go back if possible, and 86 percent said they had already made plans to go back.

78   Interview with Josephine Abalos.

79   Sofronia S. Sanchez to the Editor, "In Our Mail," *PJN* 32.3 (May– June 1963): 100; emphasis added. See also Capulong, "United States Exchange-Visitor Program for Filipino Nurses," 86.

80   "The Exchange Visitor Program Should Be Understood," *PJN* 32.3 (May–June 1963): 103.

81   Warwick Anderson, "Colonial Pathologies: American Medicine in the Philippines, 1898–1921" (Ph.D. diss., University of Pennsylvania, 1992), 332–338.

82   "The Exchange Visitor Program Should Be Understood," 103.

83   Capulong, "Appraisal of the United States Exchange-Visitor Program," 52–53.

84   Julita V. Sotejo, "Time to Evaluate Philippine Participation in the USA Exchange Visitor Nurse Programs," *ANPHI Papers* (October–December 1966): 4.

85   Garcia, "The Sense of Mission in Nursing and the Temptations against It," 70–71; emphasis added.

86   Sotejo, "Time to Evaluate Philippine Participation in the USA Exchange Visitor Nurse Programs," 4.

87   Castrence, "Challenge to the Filipino Nurses," 206.

88   Bacala, "The Trouble with Our Exchange Visitor Nurses," 136.

89   Capulong, "Appraisal of the United States Exchange-Visitor Program," 52.

90 Maribel Carceller, "Can We Have Economic Security?" *PJN* 32.6 (November–December 1963): 347–349.

91 "Exchange for Education," *American Journal of Nursing* 58.12 (December 1958): 1667.

92 American Nurses Association, International Unit to Nurses Interested in Experience in the United States, "Mailbox," *PJN* 31.4 (July–August 1962): 220, 258–259.

93 For more information on Filipino nurses in Holland, see Genara S. M. De Guzman, "Report on Holland," *PJN* 34.1 (January–February 1965): 23–27, 29, and letters from Filipino nurses in Holland featured in "In Our Mail," *PJN* 34.3 (May–June 1965): 111–113. For more information on Filipino nurses in Germany and the Netherlands, see Ida F. Lastrella, "The Filipino Nurses at the Academic Hospital, Leiden, Nederland," *PJN* 36.3 (May–June 1967): 143–147; Rosario S. Diamante, "Glimpses of Hospitals and Nursing Schools in Germany and Netherlands," *PJN* 36.5 (September–October, 1967): 249–258. Filipino nurse migration to other parts of Asia and the Middle East during this period was not as significant as that to Europe. In the 1960s, there were several hundred Filipino nurses working in Holland, Germany, and the Netherlands. In 1953, the FNA sent five Filipino nurses to work in Brunei. See *PJN* 29.1 (January–February 1960): 56. In 1966, the *PJN* published an advertisement for work in Brunei that offered gratuities on top of salaries and free transportation to Brunei: "Nurses Wanted for Brunei," *PJN* 35.6 (November–December 1966): 360. A Filipino nurse working in Turkey wrote to the *PJN* and reported that there were at least three Filipino nurses in Iran. See Magdalena Sy to Soledad Buenafe, "In Our Mail," *PJN* 36.2 (March–April 1967): 90.

94 De Guzman, "Report on Holland," 27.

95 Diamante, "Glimpses of Hospitals and Nursing Schools in Germany and Netherlands," 253.

96 J. C. Bacala, "The Holland Experiment," *PJN* 34.1 (January–February 1965): 8.

97 Manila Educational & Exchange Placement Service advertisement, *PJN* 34.5 (September–October 1965).

4. To the Point of No Return: From Exchange
Visitor to Permanent Resident

1 Interview with Rosita Macrohon, November 8, 1994, New York, NY.

2 Arjun Appadurai, *Modernity at Large: Cultural Dimensions of Globalization* (Minneapolis: University of Minnesota Press, 1996), 7.

3 John Goss and Bruce Lindquist, "Conceptualizing International Labor Migration: A Structuration Perspective," *International Migration Review* 29.2 (summer 1995): 336–337.

4 David Reimers, *Still the Golden Door: The Third World Comes to America,* 2d ed. (New York: Columbia University Press, 1992), 61–91.

5 In 1978, Congress passed a law that created a worldwide immigration cap of 290,000 and applied the preference system and 20,000 per country limit to both hemispheres.

6 The seventh preference category allotted a maximum of 6 percent of visas to refugees. In 1980, the Refugee Act separated refugee admissions from immigrant admissions.

7 Benjamin V. Cariño, "The Philippines and Southeast Asia: Historical Roots and Contemporary Linkages," in *Pacific Bridges: The New Immigration from Asia and the Pacific Islands,* ed. James T. Fawcett and Benjamin V. Cariño (Staten Island, NY: Center for Migration Studies, 1987), 309.

8 Charles B. Keely, "Philippine Migration: Internal Movements and Emigration to the U.S.," *International Migration Review* 7.2 (Summer 1973): 184.

9 Cariño, "The Philippines and Southeast Asia," 316.

10 I have arrived at the Filipino physician and nurse immigration statistics from data presented by the California Advisory Committee to the U.S. Commission on Civil Rights. See U.S. Commission on Civil Rights, *A Dream Unfulfilled: Korean and Pilipino Health Professionals in California,* Report of the California Advisory Committee prepared by Herman Sillas Jr. (Washington, DC: U.S. Commission on Civil Rights, 1975), 23, 36. See also Alfonso Mejía, Helena Pizorkí, and Erica Royston, *Physician and Nurse Migration: Analysis and Policy Implications* (Geneva: World Health Organization, 1979), 365. In their table, Mejía, Pizorkí, and Royston list the number of Filipino physician immigrants annually from 1962 to 1972. For the year 1966, they list 259 Filipino physician immigrants, whereas the number presented by the California Advisory Committee is 2. For the year 1970, they list 769 Filipino physician immigrants, whereas the number presented by the California Advisory Committee is 770. For more statistics on Filipino nurse immigrants, see Felipe Laguitan Muncada, "The Labor Migration of Philippine Nurses to the United States" (Ph.D. diss., Catholic University of America, 1995), 69.

11 National and international nursing organizations continued to participate in and to create nursing exchange programs. In 1969, the International Council of Nurses (ICN) established a nursing abroad program that enabled nurses to work or study outside of their own country through mutual agreements among participating ICN member associations. See "New ICN Program: 'Nursing Abroad,'" *PJN* 42.1 (January–March 1973): 63–64.

12 Mejía, Pizorkí, and Royston present annual statistics on Filipino exchange physicians from 1965 to 1971 and on Filipino exchange nurses from 1960 to 1973. I have arrived at the 2,040 Filipino exchange physician number by adding their statistics from the years 1966 to 1970. They offer no annual statistic for the year 1970. I am unsure if the absence of a number signifies that no exchange physicians entered the United States that year or if the data were unavailable. I have arrived at the 3,222 Filipino exchange nurse number by adding their statistics from the years 1966 to 1970. They offer no annual statistic for the year 1969 (Mejía, Pizorkí, and Royston, *Physician and Nurse Migration,* 365, 367). Asperilla also compiled Filipino exchange nurse statistics in her dissertation. Her totals differ slightly. See Purita Falgui Aspe-

rilla, "The Mobility of Filipino Nurses" (Ph.D. diss., Columbia University, 1971), 52.

13 Nalini M. Quraeshi, Zahir A. Quraeshi, and Inayat U. Mangla, *Foreign Nursing Professionals in the United States: Focus on Asian Immigration* (New Delhi: International Labour Organisation, 1992), 61. Filipino nurses received 1,521 licenses out of a total of 5,361. The Philippines not only continued to dominate the number of foreign-trained nurses in the United States through 1970, but distanced itself from other top sending countries of nurses. In 1968, 2,122 Filipino nurses received U.S. licenses in contrast to 1,288 Canadian nurses.

14 U.S. Congress, House, "Excluding Executive Officers and Managerial Personnel of Western Hemisphere Businesses from the Numerical Limitation of Western Hemisphere Immigration," 91st Congress, 2d sess., *Congressional Record* (3 March 1970), vol. 116, pt. 5, 5733; emphasis added.

15 Tereso Simbulan Tullao Jr., "Private Demand for Education and the International Flow of Human Resources: A Case of Nursing Education in the Philippines" (Ph.D. diss., Fletcher School of Law and Diplomacy, 1982), 132–133.

16 Interview with Milagros C. Rabara, March 21, 1995, New York, NY.

17 House of Travel Incorporated advertisement, *PJN* 38.1 (January–March 1969); North American Placement & Visa Services, Inc. advertisement, *PJN* 39.2 (April–June 1970).

18 Elising G. Roxas, R.N., advertisements, *PJN* 36.3 (May–June 1967) and *PJN* 36.4 (July–August 1967).

19 Michael Reese Hospital & Medical Center advertisement, *PJN* 38.3 (July–September 1969).

20 North American Placement & Visa Services, Inc. advertisement, *PJN* 39.1 (January–March 1970). This placement agency also worked with St. Barnabus Hospital in New York City.

21 Cook County Hospital advertisement, *PJN* 36.5 (September–October 1967); New York City Health & Hospitals Corporation, *PJN* 40.2 (April–June 1971).

22 Interview with Elizabeth C. Kobeckis, April 24, 1995, New York, NY.

23 Interview with Phoebe Cabotaje-Andes, February 18, 1995, South Plainfield, NJ.

24 Interview with Corazon Guillermo, May 1, 1995, New York, NY.

25 Interview with Mutya Gener, November 10, 1994, New York, NY.

26 Interview with Rosario-May P. Mayor, November 18, 1994, New York, NY.

27 Ibid.

28 Interview with Corazon Guillermo.

29 Alfredo S. Quijano, "No Brain Drain, but There Is No Job Opportunity Here for Nurses," *Examiner,* 9 November 1968, pp. 8, 29.

30 C. B. Ruiz, "Brain Drain' from the Philippines?" *PJN* 36.5 (September–October 1967): 248.

31 Maria R. Pablico, "A Survey on Attitude of Filipino Nurses towards Nursing Profession in the Philippines," *PJN* 41.3 (July–September 1972): 107–114.

Of the 147 nurses surveyed, 105 graduated from schools and colleges of nursing between 1961 and 1970, suggesting that the majority had arrived in the United States within the prior ten years before the distribution of the 1972 survey. Thus, their attitudes toward the nursing profession in the Philippines reveal the problems of the profession from the 1960s to the early 1970s.

32 Interview with Epifania O. Mercado, February 3, 1995, New York, NY.

33 Interview with Elizabeth C. Kobeckis.

34 Interview with Flocerfida F. Evangelista, November 15, 1994, New York, NY.

35 Interview with Esther Simpson, December 10, 1994, Seattle, WA.

36 Col. Winnie W. Luzon, "A Call for Unity and Action," *PJN* 39.2 (April–June 1970): 62.

37 Elizabeth Uy Eviota, *The Political Economy of Gender: Women and the Sexual Division of Labor in the Philippines* (London: Zed Books, 1992), 137.

38 Cook County Hospital advertisement, *PJN* 36.5 (September–October 1967); Michael Reese Hospital & Medical Center advertisement, *PJN* 38.3 (July–September 1969).

39 Cook County Hospital advertisement, *PJN* 36.5 (September–October 1967); Middlesex General Hospital advertisement, *PJN* 36.5 (September–October 1967).

40 New York City Health & Hospitals Corporation advertisement, *PJN* 40.2 (April–June 1971).

41 Interview with Delia Hernandez [pseudonym], February 21, 1995, New York, NY.

42 Interview with Mercedes Alcantara, July 20, 1994, New York, NY.

43 Interview with Lolita B. Compas, November 15, 1994, New York, NY; interview with Epifania O. Mercado.

44 Interview with Esther Simpson; interview with Lolita B. Compas.

45 The second preference category applied to the spouses and unmarried children of persons lawfully admitted for permanent residence. In Joyce and Hunt's 1980 study of Filipino nurses, 20 percent were married before coming to the United States. Richard E. Joyce and Chester L. Hunt, "Philippine Nurses and the Brain Drain," *Social Science Medicine* 16 (1982): 1225.

46 Interview with Phoebe Cabotaje-Andes.

47 Interview with Elizabeth C. Kobeckis.

48 Interview with Mutya Gener.

49 Interview with Phoebe Cabotaje-Andes; interview with Mutya Gener.

50 Euless Mead-Bennett and Ngozi O. Nkongho, "Staffing Suggestions on the Nursing Shortage," *Hospital Topics* 68.4 (1990): 29.

51 M. Jereos, "Supply and Demand of Nurses," *PJN* 47 (1978): 3–4, cited in Joyce and Hunt, "Philippine Nurses and the Brain Drain," 1232.

52 Muncada, "The Labor Migration of Philippine Nurses to the United States," 88–89.

53 Pablico, "A Survey on Attitude of Filipino Nurses towards Nursing Profession in the Philippines," 110.

54 Leonor Malay Aragon, "Post Basic and Post Graduate Education in Nurs-

ing: Its Actual Situation, Its Problem, and Its Future," *PJN* 44.4 (October–December 1975): 222.

55 Rosario S. Diamante, "Nursing Education in the Philippines Today," *PJN* 41.2 (April–June 1972): 39.
56 Rosario S. Diamante, "Council of Deans and Principals of Philippine Colleges and Schools of Nursing, Inc.," *PJN* 44.2 (April–June 1975): 80.
57 Perla B. Sanchez, "Association of Nursing Service Administrators," *PJN* 44.2 (April–June 1975): 85.
58 Ibid., 86–87.
59 Col. Winnie W. Luzon, "President's Report," *PJN* 41.2 (April–June 1972): 65. According to her report, a 1972 Department of Foreign Affairs memorandum announced that the EVP Committee decided "to maintain" its policy of requiring one year of service from medical and nursing graduates before they could apply to the exchange program.
60 "Rural Health Experience for New Graduates: A Must," *PJN* 42.4 (October–December 1973): 244, 246.
61 Fe M. Valdez, "Trends in Nursing," *PJN* 44.1 (January–March 1975): 20.
62 The service requirement for Filipino doctors was six months. Nursing students' rural health work experience during their baccalaureate program accounted for their shorter service requirements. However, by 1974, the mandatory health service requirement for nurse graduates increased from four to six months as well (ibid.).
63 Gary Hawes, *The Philippine State and the Marcos Regime: The Politics of Export* (Ithaca, NY: Cornell University Press, 1987), 46.
64 Manolo J. Abella, *Export of Filipino Manpower* (Manila: Institute of Labor and Manpower Studies, 1979), 7.
65 Ferdinand E. Marcos, "Address of His Excellency, President Ferdinand E. Marcos," *PJN* 43.1 (January–March 1974): 21–22; emphasis added.
66 Ibid., 22.
67 Paulino J. Garcia, "The Sense of Mission in Nursing and the Temptations against It," *PJN* 34.2 (March–April 1965): 70–71.
68 Clemente S. Gatmaitan, "Closing Address for Visiting Filipino Nurses," *PJN* 42.2 (April–June 1973): 90.
69 Fred Arnold, Urmil Minocha, and James T. Fawcett, "The Changing Face of Asian Immigration to the United States," in *Pacific Bridges: The New Immigration from Asia and the Pacific Islands,* ed. James T. Fawcett and Benjamin V. Cariño (Staten Island, NY: Center for Migration Studies, 1987), 136–139.
70 "Government Policy on Outflow of Doctors, Nurses Set," *PJN* 45.1 (January–March 1976): 27.

5. Trial and Error: Crime and Punishment in America's "Wound Culture"

1 Mark Seltzer, *Serial Killers: Death and Life in America's Wound Culture* (New York: Routledge, 1998).

2 Ibid., 21.

3 "Nurse's Story of Death Night; Names Speck as Killer of 8," *Chicago Tribune*, 6 April 1967, pp. 3, 5.

4 According to Cook County Coroner Dr. Andrew J. Toman, a preliminary autopsy showed no signs of sexual assault. Dr. Edward Kelleher, head of the Psychiatric Institute of Cook County Hospital, called the crimes a "murder-sex orgy," as he speculated that the murderer committed the crimes to fulfill a sexual need, even though there was no evidence of sexual assault. See Austin C. Wehrwein, "Survivor Says Killer of 8 Lulled Fears of Victims," *New York Times,* 16 July 1966, p. 52. In Altman and Ziporyn's book about Richard Speck, they claim that Speck raped victim Gloria Davy. See Jack Altman and Marvin Ziporyn, *Born to Raise Hell: The Untold Story of Richard Speck* (New York: Grove Press, 1967), 248–249.

5 "Headlines and Checkbooks," *Newsweek,* 1 August 1966, 76.

6 Seltzer, *Serial Killers,* 21.

7 David Halvorsen, "Throng Views Cops Remove Eight Victims," *Chicago Tribune,* 15 July 1966, p. 5.

8 M. W. Newman, "The Mass Murder: How Could It Happen?" *Chicago Daily News,* 15 July 1966, p. 3.

9 "Neighbors Sigh: 'Thank God!'" *Chicago Tribune,* 18 July 1966, p. 6.

10 Newman, "The Mass Murder: How Could It Happen?" 3.

11 Donna Gill, "Last Days of 8 Girls Pointed toward a Bright Future," *Chicago Tribune,* 15 July 1966, p. 8.

12 "Murder in Multiple," *Chicago Tribune,* 15 July 1966, p. 14.

13 Robert Gruenberg, "Jeffery Manor: Unlikely Place for Violence," *Chicago Daily News,* 14 July 1966, p. 3.

14 Altman and Ziporyn, *Born to Raise Hell,* 37.

15 "Surviving Nurse's Relatives Thankful," *Chicago Tribune,* 16 July 1966, p. 5.

16 Ibid.

17 "News Hasn't Reached Filipino Girls' Kin," *Chicago Daily News,* 15 July 1966, p. 5.

18 Robert Wiedrich, "Filipino Nurse Tells How Eight Met Their Doom," *Chicago Tribune,* 6 April 1967, p. 2.

19 William Clements, "Filipino Nurses' Heroism: They Tried to Escape Death," *Chicago Tribune,* 7 April 1967, p. 6.

20 David Halvorsen, "Detailed Account of a Terrible Crime," *Chicago Tribune,* 23 July 1966, p. 1A-2.

21 "Story of the Eight Nurses: Their Life, Their Goals," *Chicago Tribune,* 23, July 1966, p. 1A-7.

22 Judy Klemesrud, "Exchange Plan: Filipino Nurses' Role Here," *Chicago Daily News,* 15 July 1966, p. 5.

23 C. B. Ruiz, "Martyrs to a Cause," *PJN* 35.4 (July–August 1966): 196, 204.

24 Wehrwein, "Survivor Says Killer of 8 Lulled Fears of Victims," 52.

25 *New York Times,* 21 July 1966, p. 17.

26 Jack Altman and Marvin Ziporyn, "Richard Speck: The Mind of a Murderer," *Saturday Evening Post,* 1 July 1967, 31; emphasis added.

27 S. A. Buenafe, "In Memoriam: The Chicago Tragedy," *PJN* 35.5 (September–October 1966): 318.

28 Herb Lyon, "Tower Ticker," *Chicago Tribune,* 29 July 1966, p. 15.

29 Although mainstream magazines such as *Newsweek* publicized the *Post's* $25,000 offer, the public relations office of the South Chicago Community Hospital denied that such an offer was ever made. See "Headlines and Checkbooks," 76; Austin C. Wehrwein, "Counsel Advises Speck on Rights to Remain Silent," *New York Times,* 21 July 1966, p. 17.

30 Altman and Ziporyn, *Born to Raise Hell,* 243–244.

31 Ibid., 244–251.

32 Wehrwein, "Survivor Says Killer of 8 Lulled Fears of Victims," 52.

33 Wiedrich, "Filipino Nurse Tells How Eight Met Their Doom," 1.

34 John Justin Smith, "Holds Head High: Little Corazon Brave Soldier," *Chicago Daily News,* 5 April 1967, p. 1.

35 M. W. Newman and William Clements, "Senseless Slaughter: Speck Mystery Multiplies," *Chicago Daily News,* 8 April 1967, p. 17.

36 "July 14, 1966," *Chicago Tribune Magazine,* 6 July 1986, p. 29.

37 "Filipino Survivor of Grisly Murders in Chicago Lives with Nightmares," *Filipino Reporter,* 16 January 1992, p. 11. I was unable to locate published accounts that focused on Amurao's life after the Speck massacre and trial, specifically her political bid for councilor in San Luis, Batangas. During my interview with Esther Simpson on December 10, 1994 in Seattle, WA, she mentioned that Amurao's bid was successful. I thank Benjamin Tolosa for helping me confirm this information.

38 Interview with Anita Ramos Nanadiego, March 27, 1994, New York, NY.

39 Dwight Okita, "Richard Speck," in *Yellow Light: The Flowering of Asian American Arts,* ed. Amy Ling (Philadelphia: Temple University Press, 1999), 256–257. I thank Gregory Choy for bringing this play to my attention and for highlighting the fact that the Asian American woman character in the play is not named.

40 Ibid., 256.

41 Seltzer, *Serial Killers,* 4.

42 Altman and Ziporyn, *Born to Raise Hell,* 98.

43 Ibid., 228–229.

44 Ibid., 57, 62.

45 Ibid., 124.

46 Ibid., 52, 71.

47 Ibid., 129, 149–150.

48 Ibid., 206.

49 Arthur J. Seider, "The Art of Richard Speck," *Chicago Daily News,* 19 April 1967, p. 59.

50 Lawson Fusao Inada, "Bandstand," in *Before the War: Poems As They Happened* (New York: William Morrow, 1971), 98–99. I thank Gregory Choy for bringing this poem to my attention.

51 See William Wei, *The Asian American Movement* (Philadelphia: Temple University Press, 1993).

52 Thomas M. Gannon, introduction to Jack Altman and Marvin Ziporyn, *Speck: The Untold Story of a Mass Murderer* (Delavan, WI: Hallberg Publishing, 1984), 24–25.

53 Different accounts offer different sets of statistics regarding the number of respiratory arrests and related deaths at the VA Hospital during the summer of 1975. According to defense attorney Thomas O'Brien, thirty-five patients suffered from unexpected breathing failures on fifty-one occasions between July 1 and August 15, and ten of those patients died: Thomas C. O'Brien, "The V.A. Murders," *The Advocate* 28.4 (April 1985): 12. The *Detroit News* reported that fifty-six arrests had occurred and sixteen patients had died: Charlie Cain, "Hospital Probe Called Nearer," *Detroit News*, 19 October 1975. *Time* claimed that twenty-seven patients suffered respiratory arrests and that eleven of them died: "The Michigan Murders," *Time*, 22 March 1976, 47. And the *New York Times* estimated that between fifty-one and sixty-three patients suffered respiratory failure and thirteen of them died: Martin Waldron, "Trial Starts Today for Two Nurses in Michigan Hospital Deaths," *New York Times*, 1 March 1977, p. 12.

54 O'Brien, "The V.A. Murders," 12.

55 Ibid.

56 Mark Lett and Charlie Cain, "Troubled VA Hospital Calls Crisis Parley on Patient Ban," *Detroit News*, 31 August 1975.

57 O'Brien, "The V.A. Murders," 12.

58 Philip Pratt, District Judge, *Memorandum Opinion Denying Defendants' Motion to Dismiss Superseding Indictment*, 18 May 1977, 446 F. Supp. 252, 1977, 294.

59 U.S. Attorney Philip Van Dam and Assistant U.S. Attorneys Richard F. Yanko and Richard L. Delonis, "Brief in Support of Government's Response to Defendants' Motion to Dismiss Superseding Indictment," n.d., p. 1, Court File 77-cr-80149, Accession Number 21-83-245, Location Number 546152, Box 4, Vol. 3, National Archives, Chicago.

60 U.S. Attorney Philip Van Dam and Assistant U.S. Attorneys Richard F. Yanko and Richard L. Delonis, "Government's Brief in Response to Defendants' Motion for a Judgment of Acquittal," June 7, 1977, p. 8, Court File 76-cr-80884, Accession Number 21-81-220, Location Number 272612, Box 4, National Archives, Chicago.

61 Ibid., 7–8.

62 "Two Nurses Feel 'Betrayed' by Poisoning Convictions," *New York Times*, 15 July 1977, p. 20.

63 Attorneys for Filipina Narciso, Michael C. Moran and Thomas C. O'Brien, and Attorneys for Leonora Perez, Edward Stein and Laurence C. Burgess, "Brief in Support of Defendants' Motion for Judgment of Acquittal," June 3, 1977, p. 17, Court File 77-cr-80149, Accession Number 21-83-245, Location Number 546152, Box 4, Vol. 4, National Archives, Chicago.

64 Nena Hernandez, "Set for March 1: Fair Trial for Narciso, Perez?" *Ang Katipunan*, 16–28 February 1977, p. 6.

65 Moran, O'Brien, Stein, and Burgess, "Brief in Support of Defendants' Motion for Judgment of Acquittal," p. 20.

66 Richard Neely, "Deposition," October 8, 1976, p. 244, Court File 76-cr-80884, Accession Number 21-81-0220, Location Number 272609, File D-1 38, Vol. 2, National Archives, Chicago.

67 Ibid., 167–168, 273.

68 Ibid., 240–243.

69 Richard Neely, "Deposition," October 9, 1976, pp. 365–368, Court File 76-cr-80884, Accession Number 21-81-0220, Location Number 272609, File D-1 38, Vol. 3, National Archives, Chicago.

70 Quoted in Nena Hernandez, "Judge Dismisses Some Charges: 'P.I.' Narciso Declares Her Innocence," *Ang Katipunan,* 16–30 June 1977, p. 7.

71 O'Brien, "The V.A. Murders," 12.

72 Kirk Cheyfitz, "Trial to Revive VA Nightmare," *Detroit Free Press,* 22 August 1976, p. 6A.

73 "Mystery Surrounds Nurse in V.A. Deaths," *New York Times,* 23 March 1977, sec. 2, p. 4.

74 Lett and Cain, "Troubled VA Hospital Calls Crisis Parley on Patient Ban."

75 Neely, "Deposition," October 8, 1976, pp. 281–282.

76 Robert K. Wilcox, *The Mysterious Deaths at Ann Arbor* (New York: Popular Library, 1977), 22.

77 Ibid., 12, 19, 13–14, 20.

78 Ibid., 154.

79 Ibid., 166. For a critical analysis of the relationship between literary portrayals of the Asian yellow peril and U.S. policies toward Asian, specifically Chinese Americans, see William F. Wu, *The Yellow Peril: Chinese Americans in American Fiction, 1850–1940* (Hamden, CT: Archon Books, 1982).

80 Wilcox, *The Mysterious Deaths at Ann Arbor,* 161, 159, 184, 8–9.

81 Ibid., 160, 164–165.

82 Sherry Valparaiso, "Book Review: Sensationalized Reporting on V.A. Hospital Tragedy," *Ang Katipunan,* May 15–June 1, 1977, p. 5.

83 "The Michigan Murders," *Time,* 22 March 1976, 47.

84 Neely, "Deposition," October 8, 1976, pp. 300–302.

85 Ibid., 350–352.

86 Ibid., 82–83.

87 Hernandez, "Set for March 1," 6; Ann Jones, "Nurse Hunting in Michigan," *The Nation,* 3 December 1977, p. 256.

88 Assistant U.S. Attorney Mitchell Cohen, "Proceedings," June 21, 1976, Court File 76-cr-80884, Accession Number 21-81-0220, Location Number 272609, Box 4, pp. 15, 19, National Archives, Chicago.

89 Quoted in O'Brien, "The V.A. Murders," 15; emphasis added.

90 Attorneys for Filipina Narciso, Michael C. Moran and Thomas C. O'Brien, and Attorneys for Leonora Perez, Edward Stein and Laurence Burgess, "Brief in Support of Motions for Judgment of Acquittal, New Trial, and/or Mistrial," September 19, 1977, pp. 7–8, Court File 77-cr-80149, Accession Number 21-83-245, Location Number 546152, Box 4, Vol. 6, National Archives, Chicago.

91 Ibid., 25.

92   Cheyfitz, "Trial to Revive VA Nightmare," 3A, 6A.

93   Esther Simpson, "Narciso-Perez Hearing Postponed," *Ang Katipunan,* December 16–January 15, 1977, p. 8.

94   Cheyfitz, "Trial to Revive VA Nightmare," 6A.

95   Jim Graham, "Convicted Nurses Are Critical of Jury," *Detroit News,* 14 July 1977, p. 1A.

96   Cheyfitz, "Trial to Revive VA Nightmare," 3A.

97   Filipina Narciso, "Affidavit of Financial Condition," February 10, 1977, Court File 76-cr-80884, Accession Number 21-81-0220, Location Number 272612, Box 4, National Archives, Chicago.

98   For an informative history of the KDP, see Helen C. Toribio, "We Are Revolution: A Reflective History of the Union of Democratic Filipinos (KDP)," *Amerasia Journal* 24.2 (1998): 155–177.

99   Interview with Esther Simpson, December 10, 1994, Seattle, WA.

100 Ibid.

101 Ibid.

102 Interview with Milagros C. Rabara, March 21, 1995, New York, NY; interview with Priscilla L. Santayana, November 19, 1994, New York, NY.

103 Interview with Milavic D. Carroll, March 29, 1995, New York, NY; interview with Rosario T. DeGracia, December 14, 1994, Seattle, WA; Interview with Corazon Guillermo, May 1, 1995, New York, NY; interview with Hermila M. Rabe, January 27, 1995, New York, NY.

104 Interview with Esther Simpson.

105 Quoted in Simpson, "Narciso-Perez Hearing Postponed," 9.

106 *Balikbayan* refers to those Filipinos abroad who travel back to the Philippines.

107 Interview with Esther Simpson.

108 Ibid.

109 Ibid.

110 Chicago Support Group for Narciso-Perez, "'Lawyer Controversy' Obscures Narciso-Perez Defense," *Ang Katipunan,* 1–15 September 1977, pp. 7, 9.

111 KDP National Executive Board, "Genuine Support Is Needed: Intrigues against Narciso and Perez Must Stop," *Ang Katipunan,* 15–30 September 1977, p. 2.

112 Norma Deleon, "350 Pledge Support for the Nurses: Bay Area Benefit for Narciso-Perez," *Ang Katipunan,* 1–15 September 1977, p. 7.

113 "Filipino Communities Organize Support," *Ang Katipunan,* 1–15 August 1977, p. 7.

114 "We Demand Justice: Free Narciso and Perez," petition, *Ang Katipunan,* 15–30 September 1977, p. 8.

115 United States Attorney James K. Robinson, "Memorandum in Support of Motion to Dismiss," February 1, 1978, p. 11–12, Court File 77-cr-80149, Accession Number 21-83-245, Location Number 546152, Box 4, Vol. 6, National Archives, Chicago.

116 Bay Area Defense Committee for Narciso and Perez, "More Work Ahead: Narciso, Perez Win New Trial," *Ang Katipunan,* 16–31 January 1978, p. 2.

117   Robinson, "Memorandum in Support of Motion to Dismiss," 15–16.

118   Interview with Esther Simpson.

119   "Filipino Communities Organize Support," 7.

6. Conflict and Caring: Filipino Nurses Organize in the United States

1   Case profile of Elvie Santos (pseudonym), August 13, 1974, Demonstration Project for Asian Americans, Filipino American National Historical Society Archives, Seattle, WA.

2   U.S. Congress, House, "Excluding Executive Officers and Managerial Personnel of Western Hemisphere Businesses from the Numerical Limitation of Western Hemisphere Immigration," 91st Congress, 2d sess., *Congressional Record* (3 March 1970), vol. 116, pt. 5, 5730.

3   Paul Ong and Tania Azores, "The Migration and Incorporation of Filipino Nurses," in *The New Asian Immigration in Los Angeles and Global Restructuring,* ed. Paul Ong, Edna Bonacich, and Lucie Cheng (Philadelphia: Temple University Press, 1994), 175.

4   North American Placement & Visa Services, Inc. advertisement, *PJN* 39.3 (July–September 1970).

5   I have calculated these totals using Tomoji Ishi's table on temporary worker nurses admitted to the United States in "Class Conflict, the State, and Linkage: The International Migration of Nurses from the Philippines," *Berkeley Journal of Sociology* 32 (1987): 290.

6   The numerical dominance of H-1 visa nurses from the Philippines continued in the 1980s. Between 1985 and 1989, 24,417 nurses entered the United States as H-1 visa nurses. Of these, 17,727 were Filipino nurses, approximately 73 percent. See Nalini M. Quraeshi, Zahir A. Quraeshi, and Inayat U. Mangla, *Foreign Nursing Professionals in the United States: Focus on Asian Immigration* (New Delhi: International Labour Organisation, 1992), 65.

7   In 1966, Minnesota, Missouri, New Jersey, Ohio, Washington, Washington, D.C., Tennessee, and Hawai'i granted reciprocity to Filipino registered nurses. Soledad A. Buenafe, "On Reciprocity," *PJN* 35.3 (May–June 1966): 191.

8   Mildred S. Schmidt, "New York State's Experience in Licensing Foreign Educated Nurses," *NYSNA Journal* 5.3 (November 1974): 7–8.

9   Ibid.

10   "Report of the Conference, Immigration of Graduates of Foreign Nursing Schools, Bethseda, Maryland, June 23–24, 1975," Health Manpower References, DHEW Publication No. (HRA) 76-84, p. 1, CGFNS Collection, N119, Box 1, Folder 4, Boston University Special Collections.

11   Ishi, "Class Conflict, the State, and Linkage," 300.

12   Schmidt, "New York State's Experience in Licensing Foreign Educated Nurses," 12.

13 Joan McKinney, "Filipino Nurses Fight for Licenses," *Oakland Tribune,*
    12 August 1979, California Nurses Association 23.3, Carton 7, University of
    California, San Francisco Special Collections.

14 In California, Shakra observed that 90 percent of U.S.-trained nurses passed
    the state examination (ibid.). A national report indicated that in 1978, 19
    percent of foreign-trained nurses passed the examination, in contrast to 85
    percent of U.S-trained nurses. "Fourth Screening Exam for Foreign Nurses
    to Be Given April 2, 1980; Proposed New U.S. Immigration Rule to Re-
    quire Passing Exam for Preference Visa," 5 October 1979, p. 3, CGFNS
    collection, N119, Box 1, Folder 4, Boston University Special Collections.

15 McKinney, "Filipino Nurses Fight for Licenses."

16 Rosario T. Degracia to Dorothy L. Cordova, 27 February 1974, Letters/
    Communiques File, Filipino American National Historical Society Ar-
    chives, Seattle, WA.

17 Georgiana Rose Tutay, "The Dilemma of Some of Our Colleagues Abroad,"
    PJN 44.3 (July–September 1975): 150.

18 Rhea Felknor, "Trouble in Texas: Institutional Licensure for R.N.s?" *RN*
    (April 1974): 79.

19 Ibid., 80.

20 American Nurses Association, "Proposed Resolutions," 10, cited in Purita
    Falgui Asperilla, "Problems of Foreign Educated Nurses and Job Satisfac-
    tions of Filipino Nurses," 7; emphasis added.

21 J.H., "How One Foreign Nurse Organization Fights Back," *Modern Health-
    care* (May 1975): 24.

22 "Battle at ANA Convention, Resolution Discriminatory to Foreign Nurses
    Defeated," *Chicago-Philippine News,* 13–19 June 1974, p. 1, cited in Asperilla,
    "Problems of Foreign Educated Nurses," 7–8.

23 Ibid.

24 "Guidebook Issued on Qualifying Examination for Foreign Nurses Wishing
    to Immigrate to U.S.; Interested Nurses Urged to Submit Application
    Promptly," February 13, 1978, p. 3, CGFNS collection, N119, Box 1, Folder 2,
    Boston University Special Collections.

25 "New U.S. Immigration Rule Requires Passing CGFNS Exam for Preference
    Visa; Next CGFNS Exam Scheduled October 1, 1980," April 18, 1980, pp. 1–
    2, CGFNS collection, N119, Box 1, Folder 2, Boston University Special
    Collections; emphasis added.

26 Bonnie Vowell, "Why Shouldn't Foreign Nurses Pay Their Own Way?" [let-
    ter], *American Journal of Nursing* (October 1978): 1662–1663; emphasis
    added.

27 Ibid., 1663.

28 Mary Pat Colon, "Why Shouldn't Foreign Nurses Pay Their Own Way?"
    [letter], *American Journal of Nursing* (October 1978): 1663–1664.

29 Adele Herwitz, "First Annual Report to Kellogg Foundation on Progress of
    the Commission on Graduates of Foreign Nursing Schools," January 4,
    1980, pp. 7, 12, CGFNS collection, N119, Box 1, Folder 6, Boston University
    Special Collections.

30   Carmelita C. Matias to Rosario S. Diamante, "In Our Mail," *PJN* 35.4 (July–August 1966): 194.

31   G. Rose Tutay, "PNA Chapter News from Abroad," *PJN* 44.3 (July–September 1975): 191; "News from Abroad," *PJN* 45.1 (January–March 1976): 58.

32   Col. Winnie Luzon, "President's Page," *PJN* 42.2 (April–June 1973): 145; Fe M. Valdez, "Committee on Nursing Personal Report," *PJN* 45.3 (July–September 1976): 152.

33   Alicia Anloague Tupaz to Fe Valdez, "In Our Mail," *PJN* 46.1 (January–March 1977): 5.

34   Col. Winnie W. Luzon, "PNA President's Capsule Report," *PJN* 44.2 (April–June 1975): 70–74.

35   C. B. Ruiz, "Alumni News," *PJN* 41.4 (October–December 1972): 195–196.

36   Georgiana Rose C. Tutay to Fe M. Valdez, "Letters from Nurses Abroad," *PJN* 44.3 (July–September 1975): 144–145.

37   Fe M. Valdez, "Improved Professional Nursing through an Integrated Philippine Nurses Association," *PJN* 44.2 (April–June 1975): 60.

38   Steering Committee of Operation UN, "The 1965 Philippine Nurses Movement for Unity," *PJN* 35.3 (May–June 1966): 174–175.

39   Julita V. Sotejo, "Integration of Nurses," *PJN* 44.2 (April–June 1975): 125.

40   "Guiding Principles in Processing Requests for Nurses to Work in Foreign Countries," *PJN* 36.1 (January–February 1967): 38.

41   Ester A. Santos, "Resolution of Seminar on the Work Condition of Nurses in the Philippines," *PJN* 46.2 (April–June 1977): 100.

42   Fe M. Valdez to Rosamond C. Gabrielson, 2 May 1975, and C. Gabrielson to Fe M. Valdez, 12 August 1975, "In Our Mail," *PJN* 44.4 (October–December 1975): 203.

43   Tutay, "PNA Chapter News from Abroad," 191.

44   Tutay, "The Dilemma of Some of Our Colleagues Abroad," 150.

45   Minutes of Organizing Meeting, April 21, 1979, National Federation of Philippine Nurses Association [*sic*] in the United States, p. 2, Phoebe Cabotaje-Andes personal collection.

46   Core Group on the Commission on Graduates of Foreign Nursing Schools, "Foreign nurses coming to U.S. as dependents," January 5, 1977, p. 5, CGFNS collection, N119, Box 1, Folder 9, Boston University Special Collections.

47   "Fourth Screening Exam for Foreign Nurses to Be Given April 2, 1980," p. 2. Folder 2.

48   "PNA-NY Meets with NYSNA Human Rights Committee," *Philippine-American Nurse* 2.1 (spring 1984): 4–5.

49   "Technical Proposal," 1977, p. 10, CGFNS collection, N119, Box 1, Folder 14, Boston University Special Collections.

50   "Summary of Contract Report of an Investigation into the Readiness of Graduates of Foreign Nursing Schools to Meet Licensure Requirements in the United States," Department of Health, Education, and Welfare, Contract Period September 1977–March 1979, Project Director, Adele Herwitz, p. 19, CGFNS collection, N119, Box 1, Folder 5, Boston University Special

Collections. Only thirteen state boards of nursing required the CGFNS certificate of foreign nurse graduates before issuing a temporary permit to practice.

51   "Proposed Rules," *Federal Register* 45.15 (January 22, 1980): 4919.

52   "Rules and Regulations," *Federal Register* 45.75 (April 16, 1980): 25791.

53   "New Test Requirement Upsets Foreign Nurses," *Health Planning and Manpower Report,* 12 September 1979, 4.

54   Adele Herwitz, "Third Annual Report to Kellogg Foundation from the CGFNS," January 18, 1982, p. 5, CGFNS collection, N119, Box 1, Folder 6, Boston University Special Collections.

55   "New Test Requirement Upsets Foreign Nurses," 3.

56   Maria Redona Couper, letter to the author, 13 August 1995.

57   Interview with Filipinas Lowery, April 27, 1995, New York, NY.

58   For an informative history of the KDP, see Helen C. Toribio, "We Are Revolution: A Reflective History of the Union of Democratic Filipinos (KDP)," *Amerasia Journal* 24.2 (1998): 155–177.

59   "Support the H-1 Nurses, Sign Up for Justice," Petition Campaign Launched and Coordinated by the National Alliance for Fair Licensure of Foreign Nurse Graduates, n.d., Norma Watson file, Filipino American National Historical Society (FANHS) Archives, Seattle, WA.

60   "Nurses Target Cultural Bias in Licensure Exams," *Ang Katipunan,* 1–15 May 1977, p. 6.

61   McKinney, "Filipino Nurses Fight for Licenses."

62   Interview with Filipinas Lowery.

63   Bill Tamayo, "Foreign Nurses and the U.S. Nursing Crisis," *Immigration Newsletter* 10.4 (July–August 1981): 13.

64   "Extend Interim Permits for Nurses; Oppose Racist Licensure," n.d., Sue Englander personal collection.

65   "Foreign Nurses and the U.S. Nursing Crisis," National Filipino Immigrant Rights Organization (NFIRO) and National Alliance for Fair Licensure for Foreign Nurse Graduates (NAFL), n.d., Sue Englander personal collection.

66   Norma Ruspian Watson to U.S. Commission on Civil Rights, 1 May 1979, Norma Watson file, Filipino American National Historical Society (FANHS) Archives, Seattle, WA.

67   "Nurse from Philippines Files a Job-Rights Complaint on West Coast," *New York Times,* 8 April 1979, p. 41.

68   Norma Watson to President Ronald Reagan, n.d., Sue Englander personal collection.

69   Watson to U.S. Commission on Civil Rights.

70   Toribio, "We Are Revolution," 176.

71   Mark A. Stein, "Nurses, S.F. Hospital Clash over AIDS Danger," *Los Angeles Times,* 23 August 1985, Home ed., p. 3; "Hospital Sued over Child's Birth Defects," *Herald,* 1 December 1987, p. 7D; Ed I. Diokno, "AIDS Nurse Sues for $100 Million," *Philippine News,* 9–15 December 1987, p. 8; Mona Miyasato, "S.F. Hospital Death Case Grows More Bizarre," *San Francisco Chroni-*

cle, 23 June 1989, p. A8; Norma Watson and Nursing file, Filipino American National Historical Society (FANHS) Archives, Seattle, WA.

72   Rick Bonus, *Locating Filipino Americans: Ethnicity and the Cultural Politics of Space* (Philadelphia: Temple University Press, 2000), 94.

73   Interview with Phoebe Cabotaje-Andes, 16 February 1995, South Plainfield, NJ; emphasis added.

Epilogue

1   See Sylvia J. Boecker, "Professional Nurses: Nonimmigrant and Immigrant Visas," *Immigration and National Law Handbook* (Washington, DC: American Immigration Lawyers Association, 1992–1993), 280–295.

2   Jodi Wilgoren, "5 Plead Guilty to Illegally Bringing Nurses into U.S.," *Los Angeles Times,* 15 January 1998, sec. A, p. 16.

3   Rebecca Coombes, "Poaching the World," *Nursing Times,* 14 July 1999, p. 14.

4   Teo Poh Keng, "Singapore Aiming to Be Health-Care Hub," *Nikkei Weekly,* 6 April 1998, p. 18.

5   Alison Moore, "A Long Way from Home," *Nursing Standard,* 24 November 1999, p. 14.

6   Paul Ong and Tania Azores, "The Migration and Incorporation of Filipino Nurses," in *The New Asian Immigration in Los Angeles and Global Restructuring,* ed. Paul Ong, Edna Bonacich, and Lucie Cheng (Philadelphia: Temple University Press, 1994), 189–190.

7   "Visas May Ease Shortage," *Nursing Management* (February 2000): 28.

8   "R.N. Recruiters Turn to Philippines," *Filipino Reporter,* 28 June 2001, p. 19.

9   Scott Smith, "Filipino Nurses Ease Shortage," *Business Journal* (*Minneapolis/St. Paul*), 20 May 2002, Internet, accessed 28 May 2002. Available from http://www.bizjournals.com.

10   Ong and Azores, "The Migration and Incorporation of Filipino Nurses," 189–190.

11   Fidel V. Ramos, "Overseas Employment Program: An Indispensable Program," *Overseas Employment Information Series* 5.2 (December 1992): 7.

12   *The White Paper* (Philippines: Overseas Employment Program, 1995), 2.

13   Grace Chang, "The Global Trade in Filipina Workers," in *Dragon Ladies: Asian American Feminists Breathe Fire,* ed. Sonia Shah (Boston: South End Press, 1997), 135–137.

14   Cheri A. Nievera, "Filipino Nurses Will Bring Dedication, Skills to BC," *St. Louis Post-Dispatch,* 17 February 2001. I thank Dave Roediger for bringing this article to my attention.

15   For a study of Filipino home health care workers, see Charlene Tung, "The Social Reproductive Labor of Filipina Transmigrant Workers in Southern California: Caring for Those Who Provide Elderly Care" (Ph.D. diss., University of California, Irvine, 1999).

16   Sarah Henry, "Fighting Words," *Los Angeles Times Magazine,* 10 June 1990, pp. 10, 38.

17 "Nurse Court Winner," *Filipino Reporter,* 28 November 1991, p. 9.

18 Henry, "Fighting Words," 13.

19 "Platform: Should Everybody Speak English on the Job?" *Los Angeles Times,* 27 June 1994, p. B5.

20 Ed Diokno, "Medical World's 'Coolie': Federal Agencies Look into FNGS' Complaints," *Philippine News,* 3 March 1979, p. 15.

BIBLIOGRAPHY

Taped Interviews by Catherine Ceniza Choy

Josephine Abalos, March 18, 1995, New York, NY.
Donna Abendaño, January 27, 1995, New York, NY.
Luz Perez Alerta, March 13, 1995, New York, NY.
Purita F. Asperilla, November 11, 1994, New York, NY.
Ofelia M. Boado, February 6, 1995, New York, NY.
Phoebe Cabotaje-Andes, February 18, 1995, South Plainfield, NJ.
Milavic D. Carroll, March 29, 1995, New York, NY.
Lolita B. Compas, November 15, 1994, New York, NY.
Maria Vida S. Cruz, February 28, 1995, New York, NY.
Rosario T. DeGracia, December 14, 1995, Seattle, WA.
Flocerfida F. Evangelista, November 15, 1994, New York, NY.
Melencio A. Friginal, April 28, 1995, New York, NY.
Mutya Gener, November 10, 1994, New York, NY.
Corazon Guillermo, May 1, 1995, New York, NY.
Delia Hernandez [pseudonym], February 21, 1995, New York, NY.
Elizabeth C. Kobeckis, April 24, 1995, New York, NY.
Susan G. Lopez, February 20, 1995, New York, NY.
Filipinas Lowery, April 27, 1995, New York, NY.
Julieta O. Luistro, April 25, 1995, New York, NY.
Rosita R. Macrohon, November 8, 1994, New York, NY.
Fele Magdamo, January 25, 1995, New York, NY.
Irene Maghirang, April 19, 1995, New York, NY.
Mary Malecdan, November 2, 1994, New York, NY.
Rosario-May P. Mayor, November 18, 1994, New York, NY.
Linda Medina [pseudonym], July 20, 1994, New York, NY.
Luzviminda S. Micabalo, November 16, 1994, New York, NY.
Nellie Montoya [pseudonym], March 11, 1995, New York, NY.
Anita Ramos Nanadiego, March 27, 1994, New York, NY.
Rosalia V. Ordonez, May 2, 1995, New York, NY.
Milagros C. Rabara, March 21, 1995, New York, NY.
Hermila M. Rabe, January 27, 1995, New York, NY.
Ma. Concepcion A. Rugas, January 4, 1995, New York, NY.
Josefina R. Sablan, May 10, 1995, New York, NY.
Priscilla L. Santayana, November 19, 1994, New York, NY.
Esther Simpson, December 10, 1994, Seattle, WA.
Lourdes M. Sumilang, May 9, 1995, New York, NY.
Mario J. Sumilang, May 9, 1995, New York, NY.
Cora P. Van Derveer, July 22, 1994, New York, NY.
Lourdes Y. Velasco, February 6, 1995, New York, NY.

Untaped Interviews by Catherine Ceniza Choy

Mercedes Alcantara, July 20, 1994, New York, NY.
Edelisa B. Covar, July 20, 1994, New York, NY.
Christina B. Hing, February 7, 1995, New York, NY.
Epifania O. Mercado, February 3, 1995, New York, NY.

Manuscript Collections and Documents

California-Nurses Association collection, Special Collections, University of California, San Francisco.
Commission on Graduates of Foreign Nursing Schools collection, Nursing Archives, Boston University.
National Alliance for Fair Licensure of Foreign Nurse Graduates, National Filipino Immigrant Rights Organization, and miscellaneous California nursing licensure documents, Sue Englander personal collection.
National Federation of Philippine Nurses Associations in the United States, Philippine Nurses Association of America, and Philippine Nurses Association of New Jersey documents, Phoebe Cabotaje-Andes personal collection.
Norma Watson file, Nursing file, and *Filipino Student Bulletin* collection, Filipino American National Historical Society Archives, Seattle, WA.
Nurses' Interviews and Miscellaneous Nurses' Documents, Demonstration Project for Asian Americans, Filipino American National Historical Society Archives, Seattle, WA.
Philippine Nurses Association of America documents, Carmen Galang personal collection.
Philippine Nurses Association of America documents, Filipinas Lowery personal collection.
Philippine Nurses Association of America and Philippine Nurses Association of Southern California documents, Mila Velasquez personal collection.
Philippine Nurses Association of New York documents, Lolita Compas personal collection.
Records of the Bureau of Insular Affairs, U.S. National Archives, College Park, MD.

Newspapers

Ang Katipunan (Oakland, CA), 1977–1978.
Chicago Daily News, 1966, 1967.
Chicago Tribune, 1966, 1967.
Detroit Free Press, 1976.
Detroit News, 1975.
Examiner (Quezon City), 1968.

Filipino Reporter, 1991, 1992.
Los Angeles Times, 1994, 1998.
New York Times, 1966, 1977, 1979.
Nursing Standard, 1999.
Nursing Times, 1999.
Oakland (CA) Tribune, 1979.
Philippine News, 1979, 1981.
San Francisco Sunday Examiner & Chronicle, 1979.
St. Louis Post-Dispatch, 2001.

Legal Documents

Marina E. Alonzo v. Immigration and Naturalization Service, 408 F.2d 667 (1969).
Pratt, Philip, District Judge. *Memorandum Opinion Denying Defendants' Motion to Dismiss Superseding Indictment,* 18 May 1977, 446 F. Supp. 252 (1977).
———. *Memorandum Opinion and Order Denying Defendants' Motion to Suppress Testimony of Richard Neely,* 11 February 1977, 446 F. Supp. 252 (1977).
United States of America v. Filipina Narciso and Leonora Perez, File No. 76-cr-80884, Access. No. 21-81-0220, Loc. No. 272609, File No. 77-cr-80149, Access. No. 21-83-245, Loc. No. 546151, National Archives, Chicago.
Lilia B. Velasco v. Immigration and Naturalization Service, Nellie J. C. Morales v. Immigration and Naturalization Service, 386 F.2d 283 (1967).

Government Documents

U.S. Commission on Civil Rights. *A Dream Unfulfilled: Korean and Pilipino Health Professionals in California.* Report of the California Advisory Committee prepared by Herman Sillas Jr., Chairman. Washington, DC: U.S. Commission on Civil Rights, 1975.
U.S. Congress. House. "Excluding Executive Officers and Managerial Personnel of Western Hemisphere Businesses from the Numerical Limitation of Western Hemisphere Immigration." 91st Cong., 2d sess. *Congressional Record* (3 March 1970), vol. 116, pt. 5.
U.S. Congress. Senate. "Promoting the Better Understanding of the United States among the Peoples of the World and to Strengthen Cooperative International Relations." S. Rpt. 811. 80th Cong., 2d sess. *Senate Miscellaneous Reports I.* Washington, DC: Government Printing Office, 1948.

Letters

American Nurses Association, International Unit to Nurses Interested in Experience in the United States. "Mailbox." *Philippine Journal of Nursing* [hereafter *PJN*] 31.4 (July–August 1962): 220, 258–259.

Colon, Mary Pat. "Why Shouldn't Foreign Nurses Pay Their Own Way?" *American Journal of Nursing* (October 1978): 1663–1664.

Cortuna to Genara de Guzman. "In Our Mail." *PJN* 34.3 (May–June 1965): 111–112.

Couper, Maria Redona, to the author, 13 August 1995. Letter in author's possession.

Destua, Gloria A., to Genara de Guzman. "In Our Mail." *PJN* 34.3 (May–June 1965): 111.

Fabros, Yolanda, to Secretary, Filipino Nurses Association. "In Our Mail." *PJN* 34.5 (September–October 1965): 254.

Gabrielson, C., to Fe M. Valdez. "In Our Mail." *PJN* 44.4 (October–December 1975): 203.

A Group of Young Graduates to the Editor. "From the Mail Box." *PJN* 29.5 (September–October 1960): 270.

Kennedy, Fortunata T., to the author, 27 February 1995. Letter in author's possession.

Kneedler, M. D., to President Woodrow Wilson, 25 March 1913. RG 350, Box 275, File 2394-35, USNA.

Matias, Carmelita C., to Rosario S. Diamante. "In Our Mail." *PJN* 35.4 (July–August 1966): 194.

Obidos to Genara de Guzman. "In Our Mail." *PJN* 34.3 (May–June 1965): 112–113.

Rovilla to Genara de Guzman. "In Our Mail." *PJN* 34.3 (May–June 1965): 113.

Rugayan, Letecia M., to Philippine Nurses Association. "In Our Mail." *PJN* 36.4 (July–August 1967): 230.

Sanchez, Sofronia S., to the Editor. "In Our Mail." *PJN* 32.3 (May–June 1963): 100.

Sy, Magdalena, to Soledad Buenafe. "In Our Mail." *PJN* 36.2 (March–April 1967): 90.

Tupaz, Alicia Anloague, to Fe Valdez. "In Our Mail." *PJN* 46.1 (January–March 1977): 5.

Tutay, Georgiana Rose C., to Fe M. Valdez. "Letters from Nurses Abroad." *PJN* 44.3 (July–September 1975): 144–145.

Valdez, Fe M., to Rosamond C. Gabrielson. "In Our Mail." *PJN* 44.4 (October–December 1975): 203.

Vowell, Bonnie. "Why Shouldn't Foreign Nurses Pay Their Own Way?" *American Journal of Nursing* (October 1978): 1662–1663.

Watson, Norma Ruspian, to U.S. Commission on Civil Rights, 1 May 1979. Norma Watson file, Filipino American National Historical Society Archives, Seattle, Washington.

Books

Abella, Manolo J. *Export of Filipino Manpower.* Manila: Institute of Labor and Manpower Studies, 1979.

Agoncillo, Teodoro A. *History of the Filipino People*. 8th ed. Quezon City, Manila: Garotech Publishing, 1990.

Altman, Jack, and Marvin Ziporyn, *Speck: The Untold Story of a Mass Murderer*. Delavan, WI: Hallberg Publishing Corporation, 1984.

———. *Born to Raise Hell: The Untold Story of Richard Speck*. New York: Grove Press, 1967.

Alzona, Encarnacion. *The Filipino Woman: Her Social, Economic, and Political Status, 1565–1937*. Rev. ed. Manila: Benipayo Press, 1938.

———. *The Filipino Woman: Her Social, Economic, and Political Status, 1565–1933*. Manila: University of the Philippines Press, 1934.

ANA Nursing Information Bureau. *Facts about Nursing*. New York: American Nurses Association, 1946.

ANA Nursing Information Bureau. *Facts about Nursing*. New York: American Nurses Association, 1959–1961.

ANA Nursing Information Bureau. *Facts about Nursing*. New York: American Nurses Association, 1961.

ANA Nursing Information Bureau. *Facts about Nursing*. New York: American Nurses Association, 1962–1963.

ANA Nursing Information Bureau. *Facts about Nursing*. New York: American Nurses Association, 1969.

Appadurai, Arjun. *Modernity at Large: Cultural Dimensions of Globalization*. Minneapolis: University of Minnesota Press, 1996.

Arnold, David. *Colonizing the Body: State Medicine and Epidemic Disease in Nineteenth Century India*. Berkeley: University of California Press, 1993.

Bantug, Jose P. *A Short History of Medicine in the Phiippines During the Spanish Regime, 1565–1898*. Manila: Colegio Médico-Farmacéutico de Filipinas, 1953.

Bonus, Rick. *Locating Filipino Americans: Ethnicity and the Cultural Politics of Space*. Philadelphia: Temple University Press, 2000.

Bridges, Daisy Caroline. *A History of the International Council of Nurses, 1899–1964: The First Sixty-Five Years*. Philadelphia: Lippincott, 1967.

Bulosan, Carlos. *America Is in the Heart*. New York: Harcourt, Brace and Company, 1943.

Burton, Antoinette, ed. *Gender, Sexuality and Colonial Modernities*. New York: Routledge, 1999.

———. *Burdens of History: British Feminists, Indian Women, and Imperial Culture, 1865–1915*. Chapel Hill: University of North Carolina Press, 1994.

Callaway, Helen. *Gender, Culture and Empire: European Women in Colonial Nigeria*. Urbana: University of Illinois Press, 1987.

Chan, Sucheng. *Asian Americans: An Interpretive History*. Boston: Twayne Publishers, 1991.

Chaudhuri, Nupur, and Margaret Strobel, eds. *Western Women and Imperialism: Complicity and Resistance*. Bloomington: Indiana University Press, 1992.

Constantino, Renato. *The Philippines: A Past Revisited*. Vol. 1. Manila: Renato Constantino, 1975.

Dock, Lavinia L. *A History of Nursing: From the Earliest Times to the Present Day with Special Reference to the Work of the Past Thirty Years.* Vol. 4. New York: Putnam's, 1912.

Eviota, Elizabeth Uy. *The Political Economy of Gender: Women and the Sexual Division of Labor in the Philippines.* London: Zed Books, 1992.

Fawcett, James T., and Benjamin V. Cariño, eds. *Pacific Bridges: The New Immigration from Asia and the Pacific Islands.* Staten Island, NY: Center for Migration Studies, 1987.

Friday, Chris. *Organizing Asian American Labor: The Pacific Coast Canned-Salmon Industry, 1870–1942.* Philadelphia: Temple University Press, 1994.

Girón-Tupas, Anastacia. *History of Nursing in the Philippines.* Manila: University Book Supply, 1952.

Hawes, Gary. *The Philippine State and the Marcos Regime.* Ithaca, NY: Cornell University Press, 1987.

Headrick, Rita. *Colonialism, Health and Illness in French Equatorial Africa, 1885–1935.* Atlanta, GA: African Studies Association Press, 1994.

Hine, Darlene Clark. *Black Women in White: Racial Conflict and Cooperation in the Nursing Profession, 1890–1950.* Bloomington: Indiana University Press, 1989.

Hsu, Madeline. *Dreaming of Gold, Dreaming of Home: Transnationalism and Migration between the United States and South China, 1882–1943.* Stanford, CA: Stanford University Press, 2000.

Jacobson, Matthew Frye. *Barbarian Virtues: The United States Encounters Foreign Peoples at Home and Abroad, 1876–1917.* New York: Hill and Wang, 2000.

Joseph, Gilbert M., Catherine C. Legrand, and Ricardo D. Salvatore, eds. *Close Encounters of Empire: Writing the Cultural History of U.S.–Latin American Relations.* Durham, NC: Duke University Press, 1998.

Kaplan, Amy, and Donald Pease, eds. *Cultures of United States Imperialism.* Durham, NC: Duke University Press, 1993.

Lindenbaum, Shirley, and Margaret Lock, eds. *Knowledge, Power and Practice: The Anthropology of Medicine and Everyday Life.* Berkeley: University of California Press, 1993.

Lipsitz, George. *The Possessive Investment in Whiteness: How White People Profit from Identity Politics.* Philadelphia: Temple University Press, 1998.

MacLeod, Roy, and Milton Lewis, eds. *Disease, Medicine, and Empire: Perspectives on Western Medicine and the Experience of European Expansion.* London: Routledge, 1988.

Meade, Teresa, and Mark Walker, eds. *Science, Medicine, and Cultural Imperialism.* New York: St. Martin's Press, 1991.

Mejía, Alfonso, Helena Pizorkí, and Erica Royston. *Physician and Nurse Migration: Analysis and Policy Implications.* Geneva: World Health Organization, 1979.

Melendy, H. Brett. *Asians in America: Filipinos, Koreans, and East Indians.* Boston: Twayne Publishers, 1977.

Melosh, Barbara. *"The Physician's Hand": Work Culture and Conflict in American Nursing.* Philadelphia: Temple University Press, 1982.

Newman, Louise Michele. *White Women's Rights: The Racial Origins of Feminism in the United States.* New York: Oxford University Press, 1999.

Okihiro, Gary. *Common Ground: Reimaging American History.* Princeton, NJ: Princeton University Press, 2001.

——. *Margins and Mainstreams: Asians in American History and Culture.* Seattle: University of Washington Press, 1994.

Ong, Paul, Edna Bonacich, and Lucie Cheng, eds. *The New Asian Immigration in Los Angeles and Global Restructuring.* Philadelphia: Temple University Press, 1994.

Pierson, Ruth Roach, and Nupur Chaudhuri, eds. *Nation, Empire, Colony: Historicizing Gender and Race.* Bloomington: Indiana University Press, 1998.

Pratt, Mary Louise. *Imperial Eyes: Travel Writing and Transculturation.* New York: Routledge, 1992.

Quraeshi, Nalini M., Zahir A. Quraeshi, and Inayat U. Mangla. *Foreign Nursing Professionals in the United States: Focus on Asian Immigration.* New Delhi: International Labour Organisation, 1992.

Rafael, Vicente L. *White Love and Other Events in Filipino History.* Durham, NC: Duke University Press, 2000.

——, ed. *Discrepant Histories: Translocal Essays on Filipino Cultures.* Manila: Anvil Publishing, 1995.

Reimers, David M. *Still the Golden Door: The Third World Comes to America.* 2d ed. New York: Columbia University Press, 1992.

Reverby, Susan M. *Ordered to Care: The Dilemma of American Nursing, 1850–1945.* Cambridge, England: Cambridge University Press, 1987.

Rowe, John Carlos, ed. *Post-Nationalist American Studies.* Berkeley: University of California Press, 2000.

Schumacher, John N. *The Propaganda Movement 1880–1895: The Creators of a Filipino Consciousness, the Makers of Revolution.* Manila: Ateneo de Manila University Press, 1997.

Seltzer, Mark. *Serial Killers: Death and Life in America's Wound Culture.* New York: Routledge, 1998.

Shah, Sonia, ed. *Dragon Ladies: Asian American Feminists Breathe Fire.* Boston: South End Press, 1997.

Sotejo, Julita Villaruel, and Mary Vita G. Beltran-Jackson. *Learning Nursing at the Bedside: Nursing Education Practices–Past and Present.* 2d ed. Quezon City: University of the Philippines Press, 1965.

Study Committee of the Department of Labor, the Philippines. *Report on the Problem of Brain Drain in the Philippines.* Manila: Philippine Department of Labor, 1966.

Sutherland, William Alexander. *Not by Might: The Epic of the Philippines.* Las Cruces, NM: Southwest Publishing, 1953.

Takaki, Ronald. *Strangers from a Different Shore: A History of Asian Americans.* Rev. ed. Boston: Little, Brown, 1998.

——. *A Different Mirror: A History of Multicultural America.* Boston: Little, Brown, 1993.

——. *Pau Hana: Plantation Life and Labor in Hawaii.* Honolulu: University of Hawai'i Press, 1983.

Ventura, Jesse. *I Ain't Got Time to Bleed: Reworking the Body Politic from the Bottom Up.* New York: Villard, 1999.
Wei, William. *The Asian American Movement.* Philadelphia: Temple University Press, 1993.
Wexler, Laura. *Tender Violence: Domestic Visions in an Age of U.S. Imperialism.* Chapel Hill: University of North Carolina Press, 2000.
Wilcox, Robert K. *The Mysterious Deaths at Ann Arbor.* New York: Popular Library, 1977.
Wu, William F. *The Yellow Peril: Chinese Americans in American Fiction, 1850–1940.* Hamden, CT: Archon Books, 1982.

Articles and Essays

Alinea, Patria G., and Gloria B. Senador. "Leaving for Abroad? . . . Here's a Word of Caution." *PJN* 42.1 (January–March 1973): 92–94.
Allen, James P. "Recent Immigration from the Philippines and Filipino Communities in the United States." *Geographical Review* 67.2 (April 1977): 195–208.
Alvarez, Luisa A. "The President's Page: Words to Student Nurses." *PJN* 32.4 (July–August 1963): 168–169.
———. "Professional Conscience." *PJN* 29.4 (July–August 1960): 210–211.
———. "By the President." *PJN* 29.3 (May–June 1960): 132–138.
Ambrosio, D. B. "Filipino Women in U.S. Excel in Their Courses: Invade Business, Politics." *Filipino Student Bulletin, Special Filipino Women Students' Number* 5.8 (April–May 1926): 1–2.
American Nurses Association. "ANA Statement on the Practices Relating to Nurses from Abroad." *PJN* 29.2 (March–April 1960): 58–59.
Anderson, Warwick. "'Where Every Prospect Pleases and Only Man Is Vile': Laboratory Medicine as Colonial Discourse." In *Discrepant Histories: Translocal Essays on Filipino Cultures,* ed. Vicente L. Rafael, 83–112. Manila: Anvil Publishing, 1995.
Aragon, Leonor Malay. "Post Basic and Post Graduate Education in Nursing: Its Actual Situation, Its Problem and Its Future." *PJN* 44.4 (October–December 1975): 219–223.
Arbeiter, Jean S. "The Facts about Foreign Nurses." *RN* 51.9 (1988): 56–63.
Arnold, Fred, Urmil Minocha, and James T. Fawcett. "The Changing Face of Asian Immigration to the United States." In *Pacific Bridges: The New Immigration from Asia and the Pacific Islands,* ed. James T. Fawcett and Benjamin V. Cariño, 136–139. Staten Island, NY: Center for Migration Studies, 1987.
Asperilla, Purita Falgui. "Problems of Foreign Educated Nurses and Job Satisfactions of Filipino Nurses." *Academy of Nursing of the Philippines Papers* (July–September 1976): 2–13.
Bacala, J. C. "The Holland Experiment." *PJN* 34.1 (January–February 1965): 8.
———. "The Trouble with Our Exchange Visitor Nurses." *PJN* 32.3 (May–June 1963): 134–137, 142.

———. "This Issue's Personality: Juanita J. Jimenez, a Silver Lining in Our Profession." *PJN* 31.3 (May–June 1962): 192–193.

———. "The Case of Our 'Re-Placed' Constitution." *PJN* 29.3 (May–June 1960): 125.

———. "So All the Nurses May Know of Our 1960 Convention." *PJN* 29.3 (May–June 1960): 125–126.

Birkett, Dea. "The 'White Women's Burden' in the 'White Man's Grave': The Introduction of British Nurses in Colonial West Africa." In *Western Women and Imperialism: Complicity and Resistance,* ed. Nupur Chaudhuri and Margaret Strobel, 177–188. Bloomington: Indiana University Press, 1992.

Boecker, Sylvia J. "Professional Nurses: Nonimmigrant and Immigrant Visas." In *Immigration and National Law Handbook,* 280–295. Washington, DC: American Immigration Lawyers Association, 1992–1993.

Boyd, Monica. "The Changing Nature of Central and Southeast Asian Immigration to the United States: 1961–1972." *International Migration Review* 8.4 (winter 1974): 507–519.

Broadhurst, Martha Jeanne. "Knowing Our Exchange Visitors." *Nursing Outlook* 6 (April 1958): 201.

Brumberg, Joan Jacobs. "Zenanas and Girlless Villages: The Ethnology of American Evangelical Women, 1870–1910." *Journal of American History* 69 (September 1982): 347–371.

Brush, Barbara. "The Rockefeller Agenda for American/Philippine Nursing Relations." *Western Journal of Nursing Research* 17.5 (1995): 540–555.

———. " 'Exchangees' or Employees? The Exchange Visitor Program and Foreign Nurse Immigration to the United States, 1945–1990." *Nursing History Review* 1.1 (1993): 171–180.

Buenafe, Soledad A. "Some Highlights in the Development of Public Health Nursing in the Bureau of Health." *PJN* 41.3 (July–September 1972): 115–120.

———. "In Memoriam: The Chicago Tragedy." *PJN* 35.5 (September–October 1966): 317–318.

———. "On Reciprocity." *PJN* 35.3 (May–June 1966): 191.

Buenafe, Soledad A., and Patrocinio J. Montellano. "Forty Years of the Filipino Nurses' Association." *PJN* 31.5 (September–October 1962): 299–312, 348.

Calliste, Agnes. "Women of 'Exceptional Merit': Immigration of Caribbean Nurses to Canada." *Canadian Journal of Women and the Law* 6.1 (winter/spring 1993): 85–102.

Carceller, Maribel. "Can We Have Economic Security?" *PJN* 32.6 (November–December 1963): 347–349.

Cariño, Benjamin V. "The Philippines and Southeast Asia: Historical Roots and Contemporary Linkages." In *Pacific Bridges: The New Immigration from Asia and the Pacific Islands,* ed. James T. Fawcett and Benjamin V. Cariño, 305–325. Staten Island, NY: Center for Migration Studies, 1987.

Castillejos, Epifanio B. "The Exchange Visitors Program: Report and Recommendation." *PJN* 35.5 (September–October 1966): 306–307.

Castrence, Pura S. "Challenge to the Filipino Nurses." *PJN* 35.4 (July–August 1966): 205–207.

Chan, Sucheng. "Asian American Historiography." *Pacific Historical Review* 35 (1996): 363–399.

Chang, Grace. "The Global Trade in Filipina Workers." In *Dragon Ladies: Asian American Feminists Breathe Fire,* ed. Sonia Shah, 132–152. Boston: South End Press, 1997.

Cheng, Lucie, and Philip Q. Yang. "Global Interaction, Global Inequality, and Migration of the Highly Trained to the United States." *International Migration Review* 32.3 (fall 1998): 626–653.

Choy, Catherine Ceniza. "Asian American History: Reflections on Imperialism, Immigration, and 'The Body.'" *Amerasia Journal* 26.1 (2000): 119–140.

Comaroff, Jean. "The Diseased Heart of Africa: Medicine, Colonialism, and the Black Body." In *Knowledge, Power and Practice: The Anthropology of Medicine and Everyday Life,* ed. Shirley Lindenbaum and Margaret Lock, 305–329. Berkeley: University of California Press, 1993.

"Confrontation." *Newsweek,* 1 August 1966, 26.

De Guzman, Genara S. M. "Report on Holland." *PJN* 34.1 (January–February 1965): 23–27, 29.

de la Vaca, Tomas Antonio. "Should Filipino Students Take Their Basic Nursing Studies Abroad?" *Santo Tomas Nursing Journal* 1.3 (December 1962): 183–184.

Diamante, Rosario S. "Council of Deans and Principals of Philippine Colleges and Schools of Nursing, Inc." *PJN* 44.2 (April–June 1975): 77–81.

———. "Nursing Education in the Philippines Today." *PJN* 41.2 (April–June 1972): 35–42.

———. "Glimpses of Hospital and Nursing Schools in Germany and Netherlands." *PJN* 36.5 (September–October, 1967): 249–258.

Dock, Lavinia L. "Lavinia L. Dock: Self-Portrait, July 6, 1931." *Nursing Outlook* 25 (January 1977): 22–26.

"Ed. Note." *PJN* 32.1 (January–February 1963): 6.

Espiritu, Yen Le. "Colonial Oppression, Labour Importation, and Group Formation: Filipinos in the United States." *Ethnic and Racial Studies* 19.1 (January 1996): 29–48.

"Exchange for Education." *American Journal of Nursing* 58.12 (December 1958): 1666–1671.

"The Exchange Visitor Program Should Be Understood." *PJN* 32.3 (May–June 1963): 103–104.

Felknor, Rhea. "Trouble in Texas: Institutional Licensure for RNs?" *RN* (April 1974): 29, 78–80.

"Filipino Nurses Win Case: Hospital Coordinator Resigned." *PJN* 36.4 (July–August 1967): 230.

Fortney, Judith A. "International Migration of Professionals." *Population Studies* 24 (1970): 217–232.

Garcia, Paulino J. "The Sense of Mission in Nursing and the Temptations against It." *PJN* 34.2 (March–April 1965): 68–72.

Gatmaitan, Clemente S. "Closing Address for Visiting Filipino Nurses." *PJN* 42.2 (April–June 1973): 90–91.

Goss, Jon, and Bruce Lindquist. "Conceptualizing International Labor Migration: A Structuration Perspective." *International Migration Review* 29.2 (summer 1995): 317–351.

Gotanda, Neil. "Comparative Racialization: Racial Profiling and the Case of Wen Ho Lee." *UCLA Law Review* 47 (2000): 1689–1703.

"Government Policy on Outflow of Doctors, Nurses Set." *PJN* 45.1 (January–March 1976): 27.

Graham, Jim. "Convicted Nurses Are Critical of Jury." *Detroit News,* 14 July 1977, p. 1A.

"Guiding Principles in Processing Requests for Nurses to Work in Foreign Countries." *PJN* 36.1 (January–February 1967): 38.

"Headlines and Checkbooks." *Newsweek,* 1 August 1966, 76.

Henning, Janet. "Nurses from Overseas." *Modern Healthcare* (May 1975): 21–27.

———. "How One Foreign Nurse Organization Fights Back." *Modern Healthcare* (May 1975): 24.

Henry, Sarah. "Fighting Words." *Los Angeles Times Magazine,* 10 June 1990, pp. 10, 13–14, 16–19, 37–38.

"How Real Is the Nursing Shortage?" *Healthcare Bottom Line* 7.6 (July 1990): 3–4.

Ignacio, Teodora, Marlena Masaganda, and Leticia Sta. Maria. "A Study of the Graduates of the Basic Degree Program of the University of the Philippines College of Nursing Who Have Gone Abroad." *ANPHI* (October 1967): 50–68.

Ileto, Reynaldo C. "Cholera and the Origins of the American Sanitary Order in the Philippines." In *Discrepant Histories: Translocal Essays on Filipino Cultures,* ed. Vicente L. Rafael, 51–81. Manila: Anvil Publishing, 1995.

Ishi, Tomoji. "Class Conflict, the State, and Linkage: The International Migration of Nurses from the Philippines." *Berkeley Journal of Sociology* 32 (1987): 281–295.

Jacobson, Matthew Frye. "Imperial Amnesia: Teddy Roosevelt, the Philippines, and the Modern Art of Forgetting." *Radical History Review* 73 (1999): 116–127.

Jereos, M. "Supply and Demand of Nurses." *PJN* 47 (1978): 3–4.

Jones, Ann. "Nurse Hunting in Michigan." *The Nation,* 3 December 1977, 584–588.

Joyce, Richard E., and Chester L. Hunt. "Philippine Nurses and the Brain Drain." *Social Science Medicine* 16 (1982): 1223–1233.

"July 14, 1966." *Chicago Tribune Magazine,* 6 July 1986, pp. 1, 8–18, 22–23, 29.

Kanjanapan, Wilawan. "The Immigration of Asian Professionals to the United States: 1988–1990." *International Migration Review* 29.1 (spring 1995): 7–32.

Keely, Charles B. "Philippine Migration: International Movement and Immigration to the United States." *International Migration Review* 7.2 (summer 1973): 177–187.

Keng, Teo Poh. "Singapore Aiming to Be Health-Care Hub." *Nikkei Weekly,* 6 April 1998, 18.

Kramer, Paul. "Making Concessions: Race and Empire Revisited at the Philippine Exposition, St. Louis, 1901–1905." *Radical History Review* 73 (1999): 74–114.

Lastrella, Ida F. "The Filipino Nurses at the Academic Hospital, Leiden, Nederland." *PJN* 36.3 (May–June 1967): 143–147.

Liu, John M. "The Contours of Asian Professional, Technical and Kindred Work Immigration, 1965–1988." *Sociological Perspectives* 35.4 (1992): 673–704.

Liu, John, Paul Ong, and Carolyn Rosenstein. "Dual Chain Migration: Post-1965 Filipino Immigration to the U.S." *International Migration Review* 25.3 (1991): 487–513.

"Local News: 122 Young Nurses Departed to U.S." *PJN* 29.4 (July–August 1960): 267–268.

"Local News: 104 Young Nurses Off to U.S." *PJN* 29.3 (May–June 1960): 195–196.

Luzon, Col. Winnie W. "PNA President's Capsule Report." *PJN* 44.2 (April–June 1975): 70–73.

———. "President's Page." *PJN* 42.2 (April–June 1973): 84, 145.

———. "President's Report." *PJN* 41.2 (April–June 1972): 59–66.

———. "A Call for Unity and Action." *PJN* 39.2 (April–June 1970): 62.

Marcos, Ferdinand E. "Address of His Excellency, President Ferdinand E. Marcos." *PJN* 43.1 (January–March 1974): 13–23.

Marks, Shula. "What Is Colonial about Colonial Medicine? And What Has Happened to Imperialism and Health?" *Society for the Social History of Medicine* 10.2 (1997): 205–219.

Mead-Bennett, Euless, and Ngozi O. Nkongho. "Staffing Suggestions on the Nursing Shortage." *Hospital Topics* 68.4 (1990): 29–33.

"The Michigan Murders." *Time,* 22 March 1976, 47.

Montellano, Patrocinio J. "Years That Count." *PJN* 31.4 (July–August 1962): 235–236, 255–257.

Moore, Alison. "A Long Way from Home." *Nursing Standard,* 24 November 1999, pp. 14–15.

"New ICN Program: 'Nursing Abroad.'" *PJN* 42.1 (January–March 1973): 63–64.

"News from Abroad." *PJN* 45.1 (January–March 1976): 58–59.

"Nurses Wanted for Brunei." *PJN* 35.6 (November–December 1966): 360.

O'Brien, Thomas C. "The V.A. Murders." *The Advocate* 28.4 (April 1985): 12–16.

Ong, Paul, and Tania Azores. "The Migration and Incorporation of Filipino Nurses." In *The New Asian Immigration in Los Angeles and Global Restructuring,* ed. Paul Ong, Edna Bonacich, and Lucie Cheng, 164–195. Philadelphia: Temple University Press, 1994.

Ong, Paul, Edna Bonacich, and Lucie Cheng. "The Political Economy of Capitalist Restructuring and the New Asian Immigration." In *The New Asian Immigration in Los Angeles and Global Restructuring,* ed. Paul Ong, Edna Bonacich, and Lucie Cheng, 3–35. Philadelphia: Temple University Press, 1994.

Ong, Paul M., Lucie Cheng, and Leslie Evans. "Migration of Highly Educated Asians and Global Dynamics." *Asian and Pacific Migration Journal* 1.3–4 (1992): 543–567.

Ortin, Erlinda L. "The Exodus of Filipino Nurses: An Action Agenda." *Asian Migrant* 4.4 (October–December 1991): 126–129.

———. "Ethics of Brain Drain: From the Perspective of an Exporting Country." *PJN* 60.2 (April–June 1990): 10–16.

Pablico, Maria R. "A Survey on Attitude of Filipino Nurses towards Nursing Profession in the Philippines." *PJN* 41.3 (July–September 1972): 107–114.

Pizer, Christine M., Ann F. Collard, Christine E. Bishop, Sherline M. James, and Beverly Bonaparte. "Recruiting and Employing Foreign Nurse Graduates in a Large Public Hospital System." *Hospital and Health Services Administration* 39.1 (spring 1994): 31–47.

Portes, Alejandro, and József Böröcz. "Contemporary Immigration: Theoretical Perspectives on Its Determinants and Modes of Incorporation." *International Migration Review* 23.3–4 (1989): 606–630.

"PNA-NY Meets with NYSNA Human Rights Committee." *Philippine-American Nurse* 2.1 (spring 1984): 4–5.

Quijano, Alfredo S. "No Brain Drain, But There Is No Job Opportunity Here for Nurses." *Examiner,* 9 November 1968, p. 8.

Ramos, Fidel V. "Overseas Employment Program: An Indispensable Program." *Overseas Employment Information Series* 5.2 (December 1992):6–12.

"R.N. Recruiters Turn to Philippines." *Filipino Reporter,* 28 June 2001, p. 19.

"Ripe for Unity." *PJN* 29.4 (July–August 1960): 209.

Ruiz, C. B. "Alumni News." *PJN* 41.4 (October–December 1972): 195–196.

———. "'Brain Drain' from the Philippines?" *PJN* 36.5 (September–October 1967): 248.

———. "Martyrs to a Cause." *PJN* 35.4 (July–August 1966): 196, 204.

"Rural Health Experience for New Graduates: A Must." *PJN* 42.4 (October–December 1973): 246, 244.

Sacks, Karen Brodkin, and Nancy Scheper-Hughes. "Introduction." *Women's Studies* 13 (1987): 175–182.

Salman, Michael. "In Our Orientalist Imagination: Historiography and the Culture of Colonialism in the United States." *Radical History Review* 50 (1991): 221–232.

Sánchez, George J. "Race, Nation, and Culture in Recent Immigration Studies." *Journal of American Ethnic History* 18.4 (summer 1999): 66–84.

Sanchez, Perla B. "Association of Nursing Service Administrators." *PJN* 44.2 (April–June 1975): 85–87.

Santiago-Valles, Kelvin A. "'Higher Womanhood' among the 'Lower Races': Julia McNair Henry in Puerto Rico and the 'Burdens' of 1898." *Radical History Review* 73 (1999): 47–73.

Santos, Ester A. "Resolution of Seminar on the Work Condition of Nurses in the Philippines." *PJN* 46.2 (April–June 1977): 100.

Schmidt, Mildred S. "New York State's Experience in Licensing Foreign Educated Nurses." *NYSNA Journal* 5.3 (November 1974): 7–13.

Smith, Peter. "The Social Demography of Filipino Migrations Abroad." *International Migration Review* 10.3 (fall 1976): 307–353.

Smith, Scott. "Filipino Nurses Ease Shortage." *Business Journal (Minneapolis/St. Paul)*, 20 May, 2002. Internet online, accessed 28 May 2002. Available from http://www.bizjournals.com.

"So All the Nurses May Know of Our 1960 Convention." *PJN* 29.3 (May–June 1960): 182–183.

Sotejo, Julita V. "Integration of Nurses." *PJN* 44.2 (April–June 1975): 125–130.

———. "Time to Evaluate Philippine Participation in the USA Exchange Visitor Nurse Programs." *ANPHI Papers* (October–December 1966): 4, 40.

Steering Committee of Operation UN. "The 1965 Philippine Nurses Movement for Unity." *PJN* 35.3 (May–June 1966): 174–177.

Tamayo, Bill. "Foreign Nurses and the U.S. Nursing Crisis." *Immigration Newsletter* 10.4 (July–August 1981): 12–14.

Tena, Miguela Z. "The Nurses and the Nursing Profession." *PJN* 29.4 (July–August 1960): 228, 241.

Toribio, Helen C. "We Are Revolution: A Reflective History of the Union of Democratic Filipinos (KDP)." *Amerasia Journal* 24.2 (1998): 155–177.

Tutay, Georgiana Rose. "The Dilemma of Some of Our Colleagues Abroad." *PJN* 44.3 (July–September 1975): 149–150.

———. "PNA Chapter News from Abroad." *PJN* 44.3 (July–September 1975): 190–191.

Tyner, James A. "The Global Context of Gendered Labor Migration from the Philippines to the United States." *American Behavioral Scientist* 42.4 (1999): 671–689.

Valdez, Fe M. "Committee on Nursing Personal Report." *PJN* 45.3 (July–September 1976): 150–153.

"What Our Women Are Studying." *Filipino Student Bulletin, Special Filipino Women Students' Number* 5.8 (April–May 1926): 1.

———. "Improved Professional Nursing through an Integrated Philippine Nurses Association." *PJN* 44.2 (April–June 1975): 60.

———. "Trends in Nursing." *PJN* 44.1 (January–March 1975): 19–22.

Van Der Kroef, Justus M. "The U.S. and the World's Brain Drain." *International Journal of Comparative Sociology* 11.3 (1970): 220–239.

Vecoli, Rudolph J. "Comment: We Study the Present to Understand the Past." *Journal of American Ethnic History* 18.4 (summer 1999): 115–125.

"Visas May Ease Shortage." *Nursing Management* (February 2000): 28.

Wong, Sau-Ling. "Denationalization Reconsidered: Asian American Cultural Criticism at a Theoretical Crossroads." *Amerasia Journal* 21.1–2 (1995): 1–27.

Dissertations and Theses

Anderson, Warwick. "Colonial Pathologies: American Medicine in the Philippines, 1898–1921." Ph.D. diss., University of Pennsylvania, 1992.

Asperilla, Purita Falgui. "The Mobility of Filipino Nurses." Ph.D. diss., Columbia University, 1971.

Azores-Gunter, Tania Fortunata. "Status Achievement Patterns of Filipinos in the United States." Ph.D. diss., University of California, Los Angeles, 1987.

Burnam, Mary Ann Bradford. "Lavinia Lloyd Dock: An Activist in Nursing and Social Reform." Ph.D. diss., Ohio State University, 1998.

Capulong, Purificacion N. "An Appraisal of the United States Exchange-Visitor Program for Filipino Nurses." M.A. thesis, Philippine Women's University, 1965.

Muncada, Felipe Laguitan. "The Labor Migration of Philippine Nurses to the United States." Ph.D. diss., Catholic University of America, 1995.

Tullao Jr., Tereso Simbulan. "Private Demand for Education and the International Flow of Human Resources: A Case Study of Nursing Education in the Philippines." Ph.D. diss., Fletcher School of Law and Diplomacy, 1982.

Tung, Charlene. "The Social Reproductive Labor of Filipina Transmigrant Workers in Southern California: Caring for Those Who Provide Elderly Care." Ph.D. diss., University of California, Irvine, 1999.

Miscellaneous

"The Filipino Nurses' Hymn." *PJN* 31.1 (January–February 1962): 34.

Inada, Lawson Fusao. "Bandstand." In *Before the War: Poems As They Happened,* 98–99. New York: William Morrow, 1971.

Mendez, Paz Policarpio. "The Progress of the Filipino Woman during the Last Sixty Years." Paper prepared for the 60th anniversary of the First Feminist Movement in the Philippines, Centro Escolar University in the Philippines, 12 August 1965.

Okita, Dwight. "Richard Speck." In *Yellow Light: The Flowering of Asian American Arts,* ed. Amy Ling, 256–257. Philadelphia: Temple University Press, 1999.

Philippine Study Group of Minnesota. "Philippine Study Group of Minnesota Corrects the Misleading Philippine American War Plaque at the Minnesota State Capitol." Internet online, accessed 22 February 2002. Available from http://www.crcworks.org/plaque.html.

The White Paper. Philippines: Overseas Employment Program, 1995.

Catherine Ceniza Choy is Assistant Professor of American
Studies at University of Minnesota.

Library of Congress Cataloging-in-Publication Data

Choy, Catherine.
Empire of care : nursing and migration in Filipino American history /
Catherine Choy.
p. cm. — (American encounters/global interactions)
Includes bibliographical references and index.
ISBN 0-8223-3052-0 (cloth : alk. paper) — ISBN 0-8223-3089-X (pbk. :
alk. paper)
1. Nurses — Philippines. 2. Nurses, Foreign — United States. I. Title.
II. Series.
RT17.P6 C48 2003
610.73'09599–dc21   2002012388